PRAISE FOR

An Innocent, a Broad

"In her true-life tale of first-time pregnancy gone horribly awry, Leary neither sugarcoats her story nor plays martyr. It's just the facts, straightforward and satisfying."

—*Minneapolis Star Tribune*

"Equal parts heartfelt and humorous." —*People*

"Witty, engaging. . . . A poignant story with sprinklings of good old American neuroticism." —*Elle*

"If the pun of the title doesn't get you, the first page will. A devastatingly funny and poignant memoir."

—*Edmonton Journal*

"In a down-to-earth and never self-pitying manner, [Leary] recounts how she survived the ordeal and managed to laugh along the way. An entertaining, if occasionally dry, tale of a life-altering event." —*Library Journal*

"Ann Leary's account of her young family's triumph over adversity is fresh, heartfelt, and hilarious. It's like spending quality alone time with your smartest, funniest friend and learning there's even more to admire. What a broad, what a mom—what a writer. I loved this book." —Michael J. Fox

"Funny, irreverent, witty, and wise, *An Innocent, a Broad* is a story about the fragility of new motherhood and how one woman rises to the occasion big-time. Ann Leary takes no prisoners—least of all herself—in this compulsively readable book."

—Dani Shapiro

"I really wanted my second book to be sharp and funny and snide and soulful and brave and heartbreaking and true. Unfortunately, that bitch Ann Leary wrote it first. I'd hate her guts except that I want to be her best friend."

—Cynthia Kaplan, author of *Why I'm Like This*

"*An Innocent, a Broad* is always hilarious, often profound, and belongs on a special shelf next to David Sedaris's *Me Talk Pretty One Day* and, yes, even Mark Twain's *Connecticut Yankee in King Arthur's Court*."

—Ben Sherwood, author of *The Man Who Ate the 747*

"Uplifting, heart-cheering, and in the most warm and human way—very funny . . . a book that made me laugh until I snorted on one page, only to have me choking up on the next."

—Christina Barolomeo, author of *The Side of the Angels* and *Cupid and Diana*

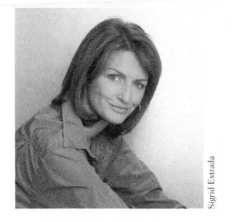

Sigrid Estrada

About the Author

ANNE LEMBECK LEARY has written for television and film. She is married to actor Denis Leary. They have two children, including a now healthy and hearty teenaged Jack, and live on a farm in Connecticut.

an
Innocent,
a
Broad

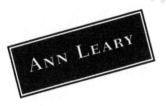

ANN LEARY

Perennial

An Imprint of HarperCollins*Publishers*

Author's Note

The events described in this book took place over thirteen years ago. In writing the book I relied solely upon my memory and the letters I wrote home to a few friends. I did not seek professional support from medical staff at University College Hospital. Any technical explanations (or technical errors) are mine.

The names of many of the people in this book have been changed to protect their privacy. Some characters are not based on any one person but are composite characters.

A hardcover edition of this book was published in 2004 by William Morrow, an imprint of HarperCollins Publishers.

HarperCollins books may be purchased for educational, business, or sales promotional use. For information please write: Special Markets Department, HarperCollins Publishers Inc., 10 East 53rd Street, New York, NY 10022.

First Perennial edition published 2005.

Designed by Chris Welch

The Library of Congress has catalogued the hardcover edition as follows:
Leary, Ann.
 An innocent, a broad / Ann Leary.—1st ed.
  p. cm.
 ISBN 0-06-052723-4
  1. Leary, Denis. 2. Leary, Ann. 3. Entertainers—United States—Biography. 4. Entertainers' spouses—United States—Biography. I. Title.
PN2287.L289667L43 2004
791'.092—dc21
[B]   2003051058

ISBN 0-06-052724-2 (pbk.)

05 06 07 08 09 ❖/RRD 10 9 8 7 6 5 4 3 2 1

PART ONE

Prom

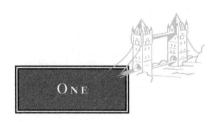

ONE

*D*URING MY PREGNANCY with Jack, my first child, I worked in my stepfather's Boston law office and spent most of the day fantasizing about my baby and about its birth. I read someplace that one should keep a journal during pregnancy, and while I've always been too lazy for journal keeping, I thought I might chronicle the labor and birth, and perhaps even send in the result to one of the maternity publications that I had recently begun to read. These magazines printed real, first-person accounts of childbirth, and I was especially fascinated by the home-birthing stories.

Who are these women? I wondered as I read one enthralling birth story after another. They scrubbed their kitchen floors and home-schooled their older children while they labored, then, when it was time to push, they pulled a plastic tub out of a closet, squatted over it, and blithely expelled a baby into the hands of an astoundingly capable husband. The children would help stitch up Mom, and the placenta would be stored in a lunch box in the freezer, presumably to be displayed annually on the child's birthday.

I admired the women in these stories for their stoicism and almost mystical strength, and I often imagined my own home birth. In my daydreams the home birth was never planned but happened almost against my will. I imagined that when I recognized the first pangs of labor, I would take a leisurely bath. Then, packing my pajamas into an overnight bag, I would realize that there was no time to make it to the hospital, and I would inform my husband in hot, gasping breaths that we would be having the baby at home. We would then spend the rest of the evening on our bed, laboring and breathing and ultimately producing a beautiful, plump baby that my husband would triumphantly slide onto my bare belly. (This fantasy would also, on occasion, include a handsome fireman who was called upon in a moment of panic.) Although I had never been able to endure a menstrual period without pain medication, I thought that with each dizzying contraction, a preternatural strength and instinctive wisdom would permeate my consciousness, and I would produce my baby with the calm efficiency of a mother cat. I also assumed that the entire birth story could be told on a single typed page.

I was wrong.

Jack's due date was July 3, 1990, but his birth story began

almost four months earlier on March 23, when my husband, Denis Leary, and I arrived in London for what was supposed to be a long weekend. Denis was scheduled to appear the following night on *Live from Paramount City*, a BBC television show that featured unknown American and British comedy acts each week. We were young and broke, and producers were not yet in the habit of flying us anywhere, but the night before we had entered the first-class lounge at the Virgin terminal as if we flew first-class all the time, and during the flight I drank eight glasses of water, just as I'd been instructed to do in *What to Expect When You're Expecting*. Our first child was due in another fourteen weeks, and I spent the entire flight basking in the knowledge that this squirming, curving, rapturous movement inside me was from our *baby*. (Even in my thoughts, the word was italicized.)

For some reason I'd always had an uneasy suspicion that I would not be able to conceive a child, and when I did, I viewed it as nothing short of a miracle. Certainly I was aware that it didn't require a lot of intellect or talent to procreate and that most people could do it. But I've always known that I desperately wanted to be a mother, and I suspected that I might be punished for some premarital sexual high jinks by having my tubes sealed shut or my womb rendered useless by some invisible disease. It's a Catholic thing. The year before, after having lived together since college, Denis and I had decided to get married, and I wanted to immediately try to have a baby. Fortunately, Denis isn't one of those bothersome types who worry about actually being able to clothe and feed the child once it's born, and he was only too happy to participate in the baby-producing scheme. We stopped using the birth control that I had always feared was pathetically uncalled for, and miraculously, after one night of trying, I became pregnant. Now my neurotic mental flight patterns were rerouted, and I was overwhelmed with fear about the well-being of my unborn baby.

I had a recurring dream as a child. My mother leaves my brother and me in the car to run into a store, and while she's gone, the car starts driving by itself. I have to jump into the front seat and steer, but my feet can't reach the brakes, and the steering wheel keeps coming off its column, so we go careening through town, barely missing fatal collisions. We keep going. We want to stop, but we can't, and then I awaken. From the moment I learned I was pregnant, I felt as if I were in that car again, being taken for a ride I couldn't control.

A near miss occurred during my first trimester, when I began "spotting," a term I had never heard before but one that's relatively self-explanatory. In a panic I left work and started driving to Mount Auburn Hospital in Cambridge, Massachusetts, where I'd been assigned by my HMO to have my prenatal care. I drove through Charlestown and on toward Cambridge on what was then known as the Prison Point Bridge. I was trying to prevent the heaving sobs in my gut from working their way to the surface.

I knew it, I thought, and as I sat in traffic, I was almost completely engulfed in self-pity when I noticed a man in a pickup truck in the next lane waving frantically at me. I stared at him, uncomprehending. He was gesturing violently at me to leave my lane and pull into the lane in front of him. I shot him an evil look and was about to proceed when at last his words sunk in.

"You're in a funeral line!" he was shouting. "You're in a friggin' funeral procession!"

I looked, and as far as I could see in front of and behind me, there were cars with their lights on and funeral-parlor flags on their antennae. I didn't remember pulling into a funeral procession. I hadn't noticed the other cars at all. Charlestown is an Irish-American neighborhood, and I realized later that the man had been admiring the funeral procession, as only the Irish can do, when he saw me brazenly penetrate its ranks.

My baby, my perceived misfortune, my swelling grief—all were completely erased from my mind in that instant, as I tried to process my newfound shame. I moved a lot as a child and was always the new student, always the out-of-sync, unwanted interloper in a group. As a result, to this day I would almost rather be flogged than find myself in the wrong place doing the wrong thing. I sheepishly smiled and waved at the man for allowing me to pull in front of him. Then I pulled out of the death lane. I drove to the hospital, where my belly was lubed and the doctor rolled the sonogram wand up and down and across my skin. I looked frantically at the monitor and saw black, white, and gray swirling lines that swelled and crashed like waves.

"Can you see anything?" I asked the doctor, not sure what a

ten-week-old fetus might look like. The doctor just frowned and kept the wand gliding around searching for something. Then she stopped.

"There," she said. "There it is."

I looked at the monitor and saw more black and gray swirls. "What is it?" I asked.

"The heartbeat," the doctor said, and she pointed to a faint light in the middle of the screen. There it was, blinking on and off like a signal from a tiny lost soul.

IT TURNED OUT that the spotting was due to normal hormonal changes, which are explained on page 344 of *What to Expect When You're Expecting*. My copy of the book automatically opens to this page even now, thirteen years later. I read *What to Expect . . .* compulsively during that pregnancy. I read nothing else. The book is made up of thousands of hypothetical questions about pregnancy, which the authors answer in soothingly matter-of-fact terms. For example, on page 138, in the chapter entitled "The Third Month," a question reads:

"I find that I'm getting a lot more headaches than ever before. Do I have to suffer with them because I can't take pain relievers?"

The authors then discuss the hormonal causes of the headaches and offer alternatives to medication, such as eating regularly and exercising. I read the book cover to cover twice before I understood why I kept reading it. It was because I was trying to find the answers to *my* questions, none of which were even mentioned in the book. I read about why pregnancy causes heartburn and indigestion, but I wanted to know how to prevent having a baby who was born with only a brain stem. Or how to guarantee that I wouldn't die in childbirth. How to ensure that my child would live a life with a minimal amount of suffering, that it wouldn't be a victim of bullies or become a prisoner of war or have a hunchback. These were the important questions, and they were nowhere to be found in the book, nor were the answers. I'm a master fretter, and I worried about every possible disastrous scenario that might endanger my precious baby—except for one! The scenario that my child might be born three months early, weighing only two pounds, six ounces, in a foreign country.

Which brings us back to March 23, 1990. We landed at Heathrow that Friday morning and were met by a friendly production assistant named Mandy and a driver named Ned. Again, Denis and I behaved as if we were constantly being met at airports by drivers and perky assistants, and on our way to the hotel, Mandy told us how excited the producers were to have Denis on the show. Tonight, she informed us, Denis could try out some material at the Comedy Store in Leicester Square, and the next night he would perform live for all of Britain on the BBC.

I tried not to think about the performances. Once, backstage at a New York comedy club, a drunken comedian had told me that performing stand-up was more difficult and unpredictable than giving birth.

"It's eighty percent luck, only twenty percent talent. Anything can happen. It's decided by the Fates, by astrology, by . . . who the fuck knows?"

These words elevated this particular comic, in my mind, from a washed-up hack to a wizened sage. No truer words had ever been spoken. Comedy, like childbirth, is sometimes just too excruciatingly painful to watch, especially if it's being performed by somebody you love. The material has been conceived with such hope and high expectations, but the delivery is fraught with peril. The audience might be too drunk to listen, or all the front tables might be occupied by non-English-speaking tourists. One mistimed word or forgotten sound effect can mutilate an otherwise hilarious bit, and one altered joke can abort a whole set.

Fortunately for Denis, the planets must have been aligned in his favor the night, weeks before, when the BBC producers had spotted him in New York at Catch A Rising Star, and they were aligned again that Friday night at the Comedy Store in London. I knew two minutes into his act that he was going to "kill." The audience hung on every word. They roared at every gag and interrupted the set with applause. I hadn't seen Denis perform in months, and I, too, laughed uncontrollably. I laughed and laughed, and our baby rolled gleefully under my ribs. I held my swollen belly in my hands and felt a delicate orb (a knee? an elbow?) glide beneath my skin, and I wept with laughter.

The next morning we had room service bring us breakfast, and we ordered up a storm. We weren't paying! We stuffed ourselves with bangers and eggs and chocolate croissants. Then we decided to go for a walk, and as we strolled hand in hand toward Oxford Street, I suddenly experienced what is technically—and ironically—called PROM, or premature rupture of membranes. In lay terms, my water broke.

It's true that at times like this we learn of what we're really made. I used to think that if I were in a major disaster—say, a plane crash or an earthquake—I would be the one to take charge. While the weak-willed people with the small brains ran shrieking into the burning wreckage, I would be the one to stop them and lead them to safety. In my mind most people were handwringers, unable to take action, while I was a doer, the one who would coolly Heimlich the choker and tourniquet the bleeder. It was easy to hold these beliefs about myself, as I had never actually been involved in any kind of real-life crisis. I identified with the heroes and heroines in literature and felt sure that I would have been able, for example, to deliver Melanie's baby in *Gone With the Wind* or rebuild a plantation with nothing but my bare hands and razor-sharp intellect. It never occurred to me that nobody sees herself as Prissy the useless slave girl, and that it's easy to feel brave when the most imminent threat is an overdue cable bill. So it came as a bit of a surprise that afternoon in central London to learn that I am, in fact, the shrieking, running-into-the-burning-wreckage type.

"Maybe you just peed your pants," Denis offered hopefully, between my wailing cries.

"No, I didn't pee my pants. THE BABY!" I screamed.

"Well, how do you know it's not pee?" Denis asked, frantically trying to wave down a cab.

"Because I still have to pee!" I cried. "It's the baby. OH, MY GOD, WE'VE LOST THE BABY!"

If this had happened on Broadway on New York's Upper West Side, I imagine that a riotous crowd would have formed. Passing women would have joined me in my panic, homeless men would have offered filthy blankets, and fights would have ensued about which hospital I should be taken to. But this was London, and while I saw that many English passersby noticed me, they quickly averted their eyes. This wasn't out of cold indifference, but was an effort to spare me *embarrassment,* a condition the British consider far worse than PROM. Any Brit worth his salt would have thought it the height of embarrassment for me to be standing on the corner of Berners and Oxford Streets with amniotic fluid running down my legs, and so wouldn't dream of calling attention to me. A cab pulled up, and as we entered, a passing, middle-aged woman whispered out of the corner of her mouth, "There's a hospital round the corner off Berners Street, dear," and then she scurried off.

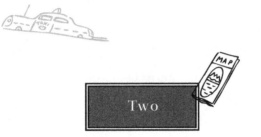

HE TAXI DROPPED us at Middlesex Hospital, and we burst through the front doors into an empty lobby.

"Where the hell is everybody?" said Denis.

"Oh, my God!" I cried. Repeatedly.

Suddenly we heard approaching footsteps, and a nurse appeared in the lobby.

"Where's the maternity ward?" I shrieked—snot, tears, and amniotic fluid flowing freely.

After an appalled silence, the nurse said, "I'm afraid you're in the wrong hospital. We have no maternity department here."

"My wife just . . . her water came out . . . and she's only six months pregnant—" Denis began.

"Not *even* six months!" I wailed.

"We're from . . . out of town," Denis said, and he said this in an imploring voice, as if he were trying to persuade the nurse to make an exception in our case.

"You need to go to University College Hospital. It's only a short distance." The nurse's initial perplexed tone had been replaced by a cheerful, commandeering one. She now spoke with the unrestrained enthusiasm of a trapped miner who sees a light ahead and tastes a breath of fresh air. "I'll ring you a taxi!"

"A taxi?" replied Denis. "That'll take too long. Can't you get us an ambulance?"

"No," said the nurse. "You're better off taking a taxi. Look, someone is being let off out front. Tell the driver you want the Women's Hospital at UCH, but it's best not to mention the bit about the leaking fluids to the driver. Well then, good luck," she chirped, and she shoved us out the door and into the awaiting taxi with great haste.

"University College Hospital," Denis shouted.

"Which building?" inquired the driver.

"I don't know," Denis said helplessly. "Is there a maternity building?"

The driver nodded, and, frowning at my teary, moaning reflection in his rearview, he wheeled away from the curb and sped through the winding gray streets of central London.

It took only a few minutes to reach UCH, but the journey allowed me just enough time to take stock of the situation and become completely unraveled. By the time we walked through the doors into the Women's Hospital at UCH, I was in an absolute frenzy and we were rushed into Labor and Delivery.

There Denis and I were told to wait in an examining room for Dr. Andrews, who appeared almost immediately. Through heaving sobs I apprised him of the situation, and Dr. Andrews ("Call me Scott," he insisted) listened patiently.

Then he said, ever so mildly, "Right. Well, before we can do anything, you need to calm down. Carrying on like this is probably the worst thing you can do for your baby, so it's absolutely essential that you stop crying."

Dr. Andrews . . . Scott spoke in such a kind yet authoritative tone that I miraculously stopped crying and waited for my next instructions. Scott said that he needed to examine me and asked me to lie back on the table. I had never had an internal examination with my husband in the room, and for that matter had never been examined by a doctor as young and handsome and casual as Scott, but I assumed the position and was distracted from the discomfort of the exam by the iron grip Denis had on my upper arm.

"Ouch. Quit it!" I hissed.

"Sorry, just another moment," said Scott.

"No, not you." I looked up at Denis and realized that the man was in a state of shock so severe that his eyes were unable to blink and his mouth was frozen in a maniacal smile.

"Three centimeters," said Scott, removing his glove. This meant nothing to Denis, who had never opened *What to Expect When You're Expecting.*

"Am I having the baby now?" I asked, sucking in a sob.

"It would be so much better if you wouldn't," Scott said.

"Although your cervix is dilated, you're not having contractions, and there appears to be plenty of amniotic fluid still surrounding the baby. You stand a very good chance of not delivering this baby for days or weeks. However, you must remain in bed."

I can't describe the relief I felt. Moments before, I'd believed I was having a miscarriage, and now I was a pregnant woman being told she needed bed rest.

"I will," I promised. "I'll lie down on the flight home, and then I'll stay in bed until the baby comes."

"Sorry, I don't think I was very clear," said Scott. "You can't leave this hospital until the baby is born. You must be monitored daily, to make sure that you haven't started contracting. Also, you are very susceptible to infection now that your membranes have ruptured, so . . ."

"We live in the United States. What if I don't have the baby for months?" I asked.

"Then you'll be very lucky indeed. But you're going to be here for months anyway, because even if the baby is born tomorrow, it'll be very ill and will be in hospital for quite some time."

Denis and I just looked at the doctor then. We were completely baffled. I had to go to work on Monday. Denis had a big college gig coming up. Our dog was staying with friends.

"So let me get this straight . . ." Denis said slowly, but then he seemed at a loss as to what to say next.

"These . . . membranes," I stammered. "Is there any chance they'll . . . heal? And then we can go home?"

"No. Well, there have been reported cases, but it's extremely rare," Scott said, and then he embarked on a rather lengthy rumination on the mysteries of the uterus and the unpredictability of its membranes. I was unable to really absorb much of what he said. Words like "amniotic" and "chorionic" were lobbed about, as well as more colorful terms like "bag of waters" and, of course, "vagina." That very morning I had awoken blissfully unaware that my womb even contained membranes, chorionic or otherwise, but now I sat staring slack-jawed at a young doctor who would not be content until I fully understood how defective mine were.

Denis spent the rest of the afternoon wheeling me from floor to floor, awaiting sonograms and the dreaded amniocentesis, a procedure I had not yet had to endure, as I was still in my twenties. I don't know if husbands are usually present during this procedure, but, based on my experience, I suggest leaving them at home. Most men I know are quite squeamish about needles, and the last thing you need at a time like this is to have to comfort somebody else. Finally, after all tests indicated that the baby was alive and healthy, I was wheeled into a private labor room, where I would be monitored for the night. A nurse offered to bring us a phone, and Denis called his family and then mine.

WHEN I MET Denis, seven years earlier, I was immediately attracted to him. There was something about his face—the generous nose, the space between the front teeth, it all worked for me—but I wasn't sure why until we started going out in public together and everybody thought we were brother and sister. We couldn't possibly have looked more alike then—I've since had my teeth fixed—and when we met . . . well, we instantly liked what we saw. During the inevitable getting-to-know-all-about-you stage of our early courtship, we learned that not only are we both Leos but we both love dogs, hate dark chocolate, are both afraid of boats, and, alarmingly, we both have mothers whose maiden name is Sullivan.

It's remarkable that we have so much in common, as our families and upbringing were nothing alike. Denis's parents were childhood sweethearts who grew up on neighboring farms in Ireland. They emigrated to America with their brothers and sisters, and they all married soon after they arrived here and settled down in the same neighborhood in Worcester, Massachusetts. Denis's brother, John, was born first, then Denis, then his sister Ann-Marie, then Betty-Ann. Denis's mother, Nora, is a teetotaler, as are most of his female relatives from that generation. Nobody in Denis's extended family had ever been divorced when Denis and I first met, but whenever anyone referred to a bad character in their area (there were plenty), Nora would say, "Well, the parents are divorced, so it's no wonder the kids are no good!"

I come from a different type of family. The divorced type. My mother met my father in college. He was two years ahead of her, so when he graduated, she dropped out to marry him. They had my brother, Paul, then me, then my sister, Meg. Because of my father's job, we moved every couple of years and I changed schools frequently. My parents were always at odds with each other. When we lived in Midland, Michigan, for example, my dad worked at Dow Chemical Company, which made Agent Orange, and my mom actively protested against the war in which it was used. When I was fourteen and we moved to Marblehead, Massachusetts, my parents divorced.

My mother was very young when she had me, and ever since I turned six, people have mistaken us for sisters, which is flattering, because she's beautiful, but now somewhat painful, because she's in her sixties. Today all my friends think she's had "work," because she looks so young, but she hasn't, and I'm following her regimen of going to bed each night with my makeup on, which she swears by.

My mother taught me to drive when I was fourteen and how to make a Bloody Mary when I was fifteen. When I was sixteen, we were at a restaurant one wintry night, and when the waitress asked what I'd like to drink, I brazenly ordered a gin and tonic. My mother was aghast, and after the waitress walked away, she admonished, "Gin is a summer drink. Next time order a nice scotch." That's the thing about my mother: She believes in good form above all else. Well, good form and the ability to make a perfect hollandaise sauce.

Denis's mother never learned to drive. She walks four miles a day, helps raise her grandchildren, and when she sees you, if she likes you, she hugs you really hard and, just when you think she's about to let you go, she gives you another little hug. The women in my family can only summon the courage for that kind of physical contact after about three cocktails. The women in Denis's family tell you what they really think—about everything. Politics, religion, your child-raising skills, your hair. The women in my family can only summon the courage for that kind of honesty after about three cocktails. Otherwise we try to say things that will make people feel good about themselves—and about us.

When Denis was in high school, his father finished their cellar with wood paneling and a bathroom, and they used to have all large family gatherings down there. I asked Denis once why they never used the upstairs rooms, and he said they're considered too nice for family and are saved for company, and I had to trust him when he said that occasionally people came to his house who were not blood relatives. The finished basement seemed a popular system in that part of Worcester, creating a sort of Irish underground railroad among Denis's relatives. Entering one of these homes on Easter Sunday, for example, you would find the living room spotless and the kitchen immaculate. Following the faint aroma of cigarettes, ham, and beer, you'd open the cellar door and find forty Irish people laughing, drinking, and eating beneath exposed water pipes and heating vents.

When Denis first brought me home to meet his family, we'd been together only a few months, and as we arrived, I was alarmed at the number of cars parked out front.

"I thought you said it was just going to be family."

"I dunno," said Denis. "Looks like my Uncle Jerry's here, and some others."

There were twenty-five others, as it was his sister's birthday, a fact that had escaped Denis when his dad invited us. We walked around the back of the house and entered through the cellar door, and there I was literally pulled into the heart of this great family. Denis's father, John, gave Denis a big hug, then grabbed me by the arm and introduced me to everyone as "Ann, whose mother's name is Sullivan."* We all sat around the longest series of card tables I have ever seen, and since I was the newcomer to the tribe, all attention was naturally focused on me. I couldn't believe how friendly everyone was, but the smiling and answering questions was exhausting, and finally I excused myself to go to the bathroom, which was conveniently located right behind my chair.

Seated on the toilet, I was enjoying a nice solitary pee when Denis's father flung open the door. Fortunately, he didn't see me, but unfortunately, he forgot something—reading material, perhaps—and walked away, leaving the door wide open.

"Occupied," I called.

*My mother's name might have been Sullivan, but the amount of Irish blood in her veins wouldn't nourish a deer tick. My heritage is predominantly German, with names like Rauschmeier and Lembeck boldly commandeering our family tree. Denis's father was a kind and loving man, and he was able to forgive me this by always referring to me as "Ann, whose mother's name is Sullivan."

I was now facing the entire extended Leary family, who were so busy eating and chatting that they didn't notice me. The bathroom door was way too far forward for me to reach, and I had about made up my mind to stand and try to pull up my pants when I heard Denis's mother scream, "For the love of God, John, ye've left the bathroom door open again!"

Then everybody stopped talking and stared at me sitting facing them—really, only a couple of feet away from them—on the toilet. I smiled nervously, and some of them smiled back, while others seemed shocked and confused. Somebody, mercifully, slammed the door shut, and so I sat there awhile. A very long while. *At some point,* I thought, *they'll have to stop discussing the fact that I'm not a natural blonde and leave the table. Then, and only then, will I leave this room.*

Between the time we met and this day in London in March, Denis's father had died, my mother and father had started second marriages, and Denis's brother and sister had begun having children of their own. I had never been the least bit sentimental about either of our families, but now, thinking about my mother's hollandaise sauce and Denis's father's paneling, I began to experience empty, hollow pangs of homesickness. Denis called his mother first, who cried and prayed, and my mother, who, with carefully controlled words in a voice she reserves for times when she is very angry or very sad, declared that she would come over as soon as we wanted her. I talked briefly with my mother and Denis's, and while we spoke, nurses came in and out of the room hooking up a fetal heart monitor, taking blood-pressure readings, and giving me a suppository. I was talking overseas, collect, so I was unable to question or protest the suppository, and to this day I have no idea what it was for. Finally it was quiet in my room, and I lay back on the bed, Denis slumped over in his chair, and we were lulled to sleep by the monitor-amplified *swish, swish, swish* of our baby's little heart.

We slept for only half an hour, and then Denis got up and raced out of the room to see what time it was. He was still scheduled to perform on the show that had brought us to London, and he was due in the studio for a sound check. Alone in the room, I was again visited by the panic that the afternoon's events had wrought. Before long I heard voices in the hallway— Denis's voice and that of a female with an Irish accent. There was talking and laughter. Then more laughter, and the two came bustling into the room grinning and chatting like lifelong friends.

"Honey, have you met Pauline?" Denis asked.

"Yes, I think it was Pauline who . . . put the suppository . . . ," I stammered.

"Up yer bum, 'twas me! And now yer lad tells me he's off to do a television show, of all things. How come I've never heard of you if yer such a big comedy star, then?"

Denis laughed and shrugged, and I was taken aback by his affability and friendliness toward this heavyset Irish woman. Normally, civil discourse with strangers is next to impossible for Denis, but since we had arrived in England, a new personality had emerged, one that was friendly and . . . well, charming.

"We'll make sure nothing happens here while you're gone," Pauline assured him, and she fluffed up my pillow and tucked my sheet around my legs.

"Just keep your hands away from my wife's ass, would you?" Denis cracked, and the two howled with laughter.

Denis left to do the show, and Pauline sat with me for a few minutes. She was in charge of me, she explained, and one other woman who was in the next room in the late stages of labor.

"This is her third baby, and she and her husband want to do most of the laboring themselves. I'll wait till they call me."

"Wait? To do what? Call the doctor?" I asked.

"No, no. She's a normal delivery. A full-term pregnancy. I shouldn't think she'll need a doctor."

"Who'll deliver her baby?"

"Well, what do you think *I'm* doin' here? Just runnin' around banging suppositories in women's bottoms?" Pauline laughed. "I'm a midwife. *I'll* deliver her baby."

"A midwife," I said, and I looked at Pauline with a newfound respect. I had never met a midwife, but I had read about them in my birthing magazines. The American midwives I'd read about were wholesome, organic types who taught women to visualize the opening of their wombs and climbed into the birthing tub with the mother when it was time to push. They were shunned by the medical community, and I took it for granted that they were mostly lesbians. Pauline explained that in the UK, and in most of Europe, midwives are trained to deliver babies and are employed by hospitals to do so. Most European women view doctors as forceps-wielding meddlers and would prefer that all their babies be delivered by midwives, and most of them are.

Pauline was soon called into the next room, and I listened to the sounds of childbirth for the first time. I had always accepted the Hollywood depiction of a woman's labor and delivery as being an accurate portrayal, and I was surprised by the lack of screaming and hysterics. There was some moaning, some long-drawn-out "Ooooooooh's," and then there was a baby crying in the next room, which caused me to cry in my room. Before long, Pauline wandered in, and I saw that she, too, had been crying.

"I never cry when the baby appears, I'm fine when the mum starts bawling, but when the dad commences with the tears, it gets me every time," she said. "Now, let me have a peek in yer knickers."

I was too astonished to protest and allowed her to pull down my underwear to examine the sanitary pad that was absorbing leaking amniotic fluid. "Good," she said. "We just need to check that there's no blood. Everything looks fine. Nurse should be bringing tea around soon. What would you like?"

"No, no tea, thanks," I said. I had been advised by *What to Expect When You're Expecting* to avoid caffeine at all costs.

"No tea?" Pauline cried, alarmed. "How are you planning to keep up yer strength if you won't have tea?"

I told her that I wasn't aware that tea provided strength.

"Aren't you hungry?" asked Pauline.

"I'm starving," I replied, gratefully.

Pauline gave me an odd look, then wandered out of the room muttering something about finding me some tea.

I'm slow so it took me a while to learn that tea is a meal in Britain. Pauline brought me an egg-salad sandwich, a cup of broth, and a cup of tea, and to this day, though I have since dined in some of the finest restaurants in Europe and the United States, I don't think I've ever tasted anything better than that tea. I hadn't realized how hungry I was, and I was thrilled when Pauline brought me a second cup of broth.

"I'm going to see if we can find you a television to watch yer comedian," Pauline said. Then she left, and I didn't see her for over an hour. When she returned, red-faced and tired looking, she had another peek at my underwear. Then she disappeared without a mention of the television. Another hour later she reappeared, wheeling an IV stand.

"I spoke to yer consultant, and he wants us to start you on medication which should help prevent you from going into labor, but it might make you a little shaky. Also, we're going to give you a shot of steroids. This is very important, because it will help the baby's lungs develop surfactant. Surfactant is the substance in a newborn's lungs which helps him breathe. A preemie's lungs usually don't have surfactant yet, so they're brittle and can collapse and cause all sorts of problems. So, God willing, the steroid will do its work and help yer little one breathe when he or she is born."

I had just started to relax, and now the talk of labor and brittle lungs had me back in a full-fledged panic. I was convinced that Tylenol and secondhand smoke posed deadly risks to my baby, and, having avoided those for almost six months, I was now being offered steroids. I cringed as Pauline inserted the IV needle, and not long after she left the room, my heart was pounding and my skin was crawling. I was wired, both physically—to the fetal heart monitor—and mentally—from the medication—and while I lay there and shook, the minutes passed, as they say, like hours and my eyes were riveted to the door in the hopes that Denis or Pauline—or anyone, for that matter—might come through to distract my fear-addled brain from morbid thoughts of steroid-damaged babies. I heard the sounds of another birth in the room next to me, and from down the hall came occasional Hollywood-style, bloodcurdling screams. I contemplated the possibility that those screams might be coming from me hours later, as I tried to push out a baby with a steroid-enlarged head.

I remembered reading the account of an American POW in Japan who was lined up with other prisoners to receive punishment for something they had done. The American watched as the men in front of him were, one by one, pulled out of the line to have their legs and arms broken with clubs. The man had to wait his turn, listening to the screams and cracking of bones, knowing that his time was coming.

I must have fallen asleep somehow, because the next thing I knew, Pauline was changing the IV bag.

"What time is it?" I asked.

"Nearly time for me to go home, thank God. It's half three."

"Did Denis call?" I asked.

"He did. I told him you were sleeping, and he said he was going back to the hotel after the show to get some sleep and would come here straightaway in the morning."

"I heard someone screaming. Is she okay?" I asked.

"She is now that she's got a big, fat, gorgeous baby in her arms. Let me look in yer knickers one more time before I leave," Pauline said, and after satisfying herself with a glance, she said, "Right then, it looks like yer going off to the antenatal ward this morning. You'll be more comfortable there. I hope yer little one waits a good long time before it arrives."

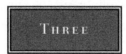

THREE

I DOZED FOR a while, and when I awoke, it was finally morning. I listened to a man speaking on a telephone outside my room.

"She had the baby at half four. A boy. Yeah, she was brilliant. Mind you, she labored for eleven hours, so she's a bit knackered."

Although I was in a tiny room with no view, everything, even the air, was foreign and strange, and I wished for the millionth time that I had been in Boston or New York during my PROM.

Before that weekend I'd had relatively little experience with the English as a people. I had no close friends who were English, but when I was in college I had waitressed at a restaurant called the Boston Brewery, which brewed its own English-style beer. At that time the restaurant/brewery was a fading trend, and the owner, a British millionaire named Simon, blamed his employees for his restaurant's troubles and berated us constantly.

"Where," he would ask the restaurant manager at a staff meeting, "did you receive your management training?"

The manager would think long and hard and then reply, "I guess, working in restaurants."

"Working in restaurants," Simon would sneer, shaking his head in disbelief. "No management training or business education of any kind, eh? Well, I must say I'm not surprised."

Then he would proceed to the humbling of us lowlier wage earners.

"Only in America," he'd exclaim, "do waiters believe that they deserve tips regardless of the quality of service! But that's the American work ethic for you, isn't it?"

Citing breaches in restaurant protocol and check-adding errors, he called us lazy and stupid. He marveled at the inadequacies of the American educational system, which turned out individuals like us, who lacked even rudimentary math skills and had not the vaguest knowledge of the world outside the United States.

Inevitably one of the dishwashers would mutter under his breath, "Anytime you want to thank us for bailing out your ass in World War Two is fine with me," and we'd all snort with laughter.

A busboy would whisper, "I think you Limeys were singing a different tune when we kicked your ass in the Revolutionary War," and we would choke with mirth.

We received the owner's slurs with an attitude of bemused pity, having been raised to believe that we Americans are mentally, physically, and spiritually superior to all other people and that any foreigner who says otherwise must be consumed with bitter jealousy. Simon's relatively refined English mannerisms confirmed for most of the staff what his accent had already made us suspect—the man was gay, and his constant references to his wife and daughter in Britain were viewed with skepticism.

"Whatta ya expect from a guy whose country is run by a queen nobody even voted for?" I heard the bartender once say to a waiter, and the waiter nodded gravely in agreement.

I assumed that the English who now surrounded me shared my former boss's views that Americans are slothful and stupid, and I was determined to prove myself an exception to the rule. When a pair of young doctors entered my room early that morning and nodded at me, I tried to look intelligent, but that's a difficult task for somebody whose leaking body is confined to a bed. I had nothing to read or even to look at, so I narrowed my eyes and stared at my fingernails, in what I hoped was a thoughtful way. Then I glanced at the doctors, who were examining a chart that hung from a clipboard at the end of my bed. One of them smiled and nodded, I returned my gaze to my fingernails, and they left the room.

Sometime later Scott entered the room accompanied by the two other young doctors, and I was terribly relieved to see a familiar face.

"Good morning," said Scott.

"Hi," I bleated. I was suddenly almost mute with shyness and was forced to abandon any pretense of intelligence.

"This is Nigel, and this is Jeff. They're residents. How did you do last night?"

"Fine," I croaked.

Scott lifted the clipboard off my bed and frowned at the chart.

"I'm . . . a little worried about all the medication and the effect it might have on the baby," I whined.

"Well, that's a legitimate concern," said Scott. "But these medications have been used for years. Their benefits far out-weigh any risks to you and your baby. Anyway, we're taking you off the drip, and you'll only need one more shot of the betamethasone, the steroid, and then you're finished with that as well."

The two residents were looking at my chart with Scott.

"She arrived under the impression that the baby was twenty-five weeks' gestation, but the scan reveals a baby which appears to be closer to twenty-six weeks," Scott said to them.

"Ah, so *this* is the American woman," Nigel said, and Scott nodded, leaving me to speculate on the nature of the morning's staff meeting. I imagined Scott's wry and witty account of our hapless arrival, including a warning to the staff about our igno-rance and about the fact that I had not had a bikini wax in some time.

"Right then," said Scott. "You'll be moving up to the antenatal ward as soon as we can get one of the sisters to help you. We're doing rounds up there later this morning, so we'll see you then."

About an hour later, a short blond girl arrived with a wheelchair. "Good morning, Mrs. Leary. I'm Celia," she said in an impossibly quiet voice. "Are you ready to move to the antenatal ward?"

"Okay, but I'm worried that my husband won't be able to find me. Will somebody tell him where I am?"

"Of course," Celia whispered. "We don't want him to find the empty bed here and think . . ." Her faint voice tapered off then, or at least I could no longer hear it. She motioned toward the wheelchair. "Please slide out of the bed and carefully sit in the chair. You're not to move around very much, I'm afraid."

As I slid into the wheelchair, I noticed that Celia's name tag said SISTER CECELIA OSGOOD. She was young and shy and pretty and unlike any of the nuns I had ever known. Last night Pauline had made reference to one of the "sisters" on duty, and I began to wonder if we had happened upon a Catholic hospital here in the middle of London. But, since it lacked the name of a saint, that seemed unlikely. An administrator had asked me my religion when we were admitted, and I'd said Catholic, although Denis and I never went to church. Perhaps they liked to have nuns care for the Catholic people in the hospital, I thought, and my next deluded, anxiety-ridden thought was that perhaps in retaliation for the acts of the IRA, Irish Catholics were segregated in the hospital and treated by nuns instead of proper nurses.

We rode the elevator to the third floor, and Sister Celia wheeled me down a hall and into a large room at the end. It was brightly lit, due to the high windows, which were cranked open that warm March morning. Beds lined the walls of the room— eight, crowded close together—and although most were rumpled and cluttered with personal belongings, only one of the beds had a patient in it. The rest of the beds' occupants sat around a long table in the middle of the floor, eating breakfast. Celia pushed me past the table, and the women, all of them pregnant, stopped talking. I noticed several surreptitious glances and was immediately conscious of my hospital-issue gown, a flimsy smock that was open in the back. A hole lay where the fastener had once been located, and I clutched the garment around me as I climbed from the wheelchair into one of the beds. The women at the table wore real nightgowns and robes with matching slippers. They had obviously packed for their stay, and from their sizes I could see that they were all further along in their pregnancies than I was.

It occurred to me that I hadn't seen myself in a mirror since the morning before. Running my fingers through my short hair, I discovered that it stood up on one side and could not be persuaded to lie flat. My bed faced the table, and the women were now talking quietly among themselves. I noticed one young woman glance at me, then whisper to the very pretty young woman next to her, who giggled. Did I mention that I moved a lot as a kid? Suddenly I felt like a new student being offered to the most popular clique for their endorsement.

It had never occurred to me that in my late twenties I would find myself again in a position where my clothes and accent might be reason for ostracism, but here I was, pulling my sheet up over my gown and staring at the ceiling. When Sister Celia asked if I would like anything else, I smiled and shook my head, determined that the room's occupants not learn I was an American.

The women at the table finished their breakfasts, and a few returned to their beds. The rest filed out of the room, chatting amiably. In the bed on my left was a woman who had been asleep when I arrived. Now she was awake and reading a book. On my right was a young, round-faced woman who had been one of the more talkative at the breakfast table and, in my regressing, fifth-grader's mind, the most popular. From the accumulation of belongings on and around her bed, it looked like she'd been in the ward for some time, and I saw her arrange little gift bunnies and bears around her.

I had to use the bathroom. In the labor ward, I had been forced to use a bedpan. Could it be possible that I was expected to do the same thing here, in the presence of others? I didn't see any bedpans, but I was afraid to stand up. After what seemed an eternity, a nurse walked into the room and past my bed.

"Excuse me," I said softly. My face reddened at the sound of my voice, but the nurse walked on, unable to hear my timid call.

"OY!" bellowed the round-faced girl next to me. The nurse stopped in her tracks.

"She wants sumfin, don't she?" the girl said, nodding in my direction.

"Yes, Mrs. Leary?" the nurse said.

"I have to go to the bathroom," I whispered.

"Well, go ahead then," the nurse replied.

"Okay," I said. "I wasn't sure if I was still on bed rest."

"You are," said the nurse, impatiently, "but you're allowed to get up to use the loo, for heaven's sake. Go on, it's right outside the ward."

When I got back to my bed, the other women were returning from wherever they had gone, and they were also settling into their beds. I noticed that each bed had next to it a chair and a table, which contained three drawers. A housekeeper was mopping the floor. Another housekeeper was changing sheets. She went from bed to bed, and each bed's occupant sat on her chair until she was finished. I looked longingly at the book that my neighbor was reading. I need to read on the toilet, in traffic, in line at the deli. My own thoughts have never been interesting or entertaining, but for the past eighteen hours, I had been forced to endure them. I started to make a mental note of what I wanted Denis to bring me, books, magazines, and newspapers being at the top of the list.

"Are you American?"

The round-faced girl was leaning on the side of her bed facing me. I saw now that her belly was enormous.

"Yes," I said, trying to flatten my hair.

"I thought so," she said, then turning around, she said to the girl in the bed behind her, "There, you stewpid cow, I told you she's not Australian."

"Shut up, Sophie, I'm trying to read me horoscope," her neighbor replied with a smirk.

"Read mine. Virgo," Sophie said.

"Virgo?" said her neighbor.

"Yeah, that's right. The virgin, that's me," laughed Sophie, and her neighbor read her a horoscope that assured success in the workplace and alluded to a romantic encounter in the next few days.

"That must mean the baby comes today, then," Sophie said, and turning to me she asked, "When's yours due?"

"July third."

"Most of us is in here 'cuz we're overdue now. My baby was due ten days ago. There was a girl here who was trying to keep from having a premature baby, but she had the baby Friday. Baby's in the Special Care Baby Unit now. I hear he's doing awright. Joan, you was brought in for premature labor, right?"

"Yes," replied the woman on my left. I turned to look at her, and she put down her book. "Hello," she said. "I'm Joan Finch."

"Hi, I'm Ann Leary."

Joan was in her thirty-first week of pregnancy; her membranes had ruptured earlier at twenty-seven weeks. She lived in the London suburbs, she told me, but had been transferred to UCH because the neonatal unit was superior to the one in her area. Joan was kind and soft-spoken and appeared to be approximately the same age as I was, while Sophie and some of the others looked like teenagers. When I told Joan how I came to be at UCH, she commiserated kindly, and I was just thinking

how lucky I was to have a neighbor like Joan when she
informed me that she would be leaving UCH later in the week.
Once she reached thirty-two weeks' gestation, she could return
to her local hospital for the remainder of her pregnancy.

Joan went back to her book. Sophie was now seated on the
bed across from me, talking with the pretty girl I had noticed at
the breakfast table. They chatted quietly and giggled, and
although I tried to tell myself it didn't matter, I was convinced
they were talking about me, about my bad hair and my accent
and my sadly insufficient girth.

Finally Denis arrived, dressed in yesterday's clothes and
reeking of cigarettes. He seemed slightly taken aback by the
presence of so many other women in nighties, and he pulled a
chair up close to my bed and kissed me self-consciously.

"Where have you been?" I whispered angrily.

"I just woke up," he replied. "It's nine o'clock in the morning.
They don't allow visitors until now."

"Nine o'clock? I feel like I've been in this bed for months."

"How's the baby?" Denis asked.

"Shhhh!"

"What?"

"I don't think everybody has to hear everything we say, if
that's all right with you," I whispered.

Denis looked around. "There's a curtain here. We can pull it
around the bed if you want some privacy."

"No!" I hissed.

"Jesus, why not?"

"Nobody else has their curtain closed. They'll think we have an attitude."

"That's ridiculous," Denis said, rising to close the curtain. I grabbed his pant leg.

"Please," I begged. "Please don't close it. . . ."

Denis sat back down. "All right. I don't see why it's such a big deal."

A young man walked in, and as he passed us, he said to Denis, "You found her all right?"

"Yeah. Thanks, man," Denis replied.

"Cheers," the man said, and then he walked over to where Sophie sat with the other girl.

"Who's that?" I murmured to Denis.

"I met him in the smoking room. His girlfriend's up here. I guess that's her."

"Hmmm," I said.

"How are you feeling? Is the baby moving and everything?"

"Yeah," I said.

"Good," Denis said. Then he leaned in close. "The show went really well. I mean, *really* well. The audience went nuts, but the weirdest thing is that I got stopped twice on the way over here—by people on the street who recognized me from the show. Amazing, huh?"

I looked at him then, truly amazed.

"It turns out there are only four channels that most people get here, and that's kind of the only show to watch on Saturday nights, so a lot of people saw it—"

"Are you out of your mind?" I said under my breath.

"What?"

"Do you think I care about your set? Look at me. I'm sitting in what is essentially my new home for possibly the next three months, with roommates who hate me, carrying a baby who might *die,* and I'm supposed to be excited about some stupid comedy show?"

"No, I didn't . . . your roommates hate you already?" Denis asked.

"I'm pretty sure," I said. "Anyway, I thought you might come back last night."

"I was going to," he replied, "but I called, and that nurse told me you were asleep. So I went to this . . . thing . . . and then back to the hotel."

"What kind of *thing?*"

"It was a party. Somebody from the show invited me, you know, so I felt like I had to go."

"Oh," I said. It did seem silly to expect Denis to go back to his room and fret about me, when there was nothing he could do for me anyway. I imagined him sitting alone at the bar wherever this party was, pouring his troubles out to a sympathetic bartender.

"Hey, I almost forgot to tell you!" exclaimed Denis. "Joe Strummer was there and it turns out he and his wife had a premature baby right here at UCH a few years ago and—"

"Joe Strummer? Joe Strummer, from the Clash, was at the party?"

"Yeah, his kid's fine now, but he was telling me some stuff about the doctors here and . . ."

Denis's lips were moving but I couldn't hear what he was saying. I was too busy picturing him in the center of a boisterous crowd, being toasted by Mick Jagger and Jerry Hall. Keith Richards and Elton John were tugging at his sleeves trying to get his attention, and photographers from *HELLO!* and *OK!* were fighting each other to get his picture. At the end of the evening, in my newly caustic mind, it was Naomi Campbell lending Denis a sympathetic ear, and I was seized with jealousy and rage.

"I just don't understand how you could go to a party and have the time of your life with a bunch of celebrities while your wife and baby are trying NOT TO DIE!"

"Shhhh!" Denis whispered. "Now *you're* talking too loud!"

Thrilled with the opportunity to escape my bitter hospital bed, Denis went out and bought me some books and magazines and brought me my things from the hotel so that I could finally brush my teeth and hair. The other girls had visitors, quite a lot as it was Sunday, and Denis and I spent the afternoon eavesdropping on their conversations, playing gin rummy, and drinking a revolting soft drink called Lucozade. At six it was time for visitors to leave. Denis had gotten himself booked at the Comedy Store. He could stay one more night in our hotel, and then he had to find a cheaper place.

That evening at supper, all the girls got up and sat around the table, which the housekeeper had set up for dinner. I remained in my bed as the housekeeper brought in the trays of food.

"Yer not sitting at the table?" the housekeeper asked.

"I don't think I am supposed to . . . ," I began, but the housekeeper handed me my tray and served the others at the table. I ate my supper while staring at a Jeffrey Archer paperback that Denis had brought me. I had just discovered that, in addition to my other problems, I was now unable to read. I looked at the pages but was able to absorb only one or two words before my thoughts would veer from the book to my frantic fears and misgivings. *Will the baby live? Will it be normal? Do the other women think I'm a snob for not sitting at the table with them? Will the baby live? Why did I get on that airplane? Why did I come? Does everybody in this ward understand that I'm on bed rest?*

"What are you reading? *Ralph Nader's Consumer's Guide to Hospitals in the UK?*"

I was startled by the man's voice and looked up to see a blond man, fortyish, wearing a tuxedo.

"Ummm . . . ," I replied.

"Maxwell Prosser. I'm your consultant. I was going to meet you tomorrow, but I had to look in on another patient, so I thought I'd see how you're getting on."

"Oh, okay," I replied.

I had been told by the nurses that they were talking to my "consultant," Mr. Prosser, about me, and I assumed that this Mr. Prosser was a hospital administrator. The British use of the term "Mr." for surgeons, I later learned, dates back to the Middle Ages, when surgeons belonged to the same guild as barbers and were described as "barber surgeons." By the eighteenth century, there were three types of medical "professionals"—physicians, surgeons, and apothecaries. Of these, physicians ranked highest in status, apothecaries lowest. Physicians were educated in universities and were required to qualify for a degree. They were addressed as doctors but were never trained in surgery and never allowed to "cut" patients. Surgeons did not receive a degree from a university. Instead they served as apprentices to other surgeons, and when their apprenticeship was over, they took an examination. If they passed, they were awarded a diploma, not a degree, and were therefore unable to call themselves doctors and were referred to as "Mr."

Of course, today both doctors and surgeons must attend medical school to receive their degrees. If a doctor chooses to become a surgeon, he is required to receive further postgraduate training before he can become a consultant surgeon. So, in effect, my consultant began his career as Mr. Prosser, became Dr. Prosser, and, upon reaching consultant status, became Mr. Prosser again.

Apparently I was staring at Mr. Prosser's dinner jacket as he said, dryly, "I always dress like this when tending American patients." Then he lifted the chart off my bed and stared at it for a moment.

"Right," he said. "I'm afraid I've got my wife waiting in the car. We're going to a charity event, but I'll give you the quick rundown. A full-term pregnancy lasts forty weeks. Your membranes ruptured at twenty-six weeks. That's too early. If your baby were to be born today or tomorrow, it would only have about a fifty percent chance of survival. We're going to try to keep you from having the baby as long as we can. A baby born at twenty-seven weeks is better than a baby born at twenty-six weeks. A baby born at thirty weeks is even better. Once a baby reaches thirty-two weeks, its survival rate is excellent, and our goal is to get you to at least thirty-two weeks."

My mind was swimming. "But if the baby's born in the next few days . . . ," I started.

"The baby will be very ill."

Amazingly, I found Mr. Prosser's forthright British manner comforting. The information he was conveying was devastating, but his no-nonsense delivery, his dry humor, and his formal attire gave him an air of such authority that it was impossible to imagine a baby's having the audacity to be born before Mr. Prosser said it was okay. Mr. Prosser said he'd check in during rounds tomorrow, and then he was gone.

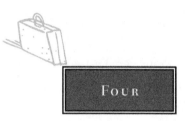

Four

$\mathcal{B}$EFORE I WAS admitted to University College Hospital, my knowledge of Britain's National Health Service was almost nonexistent. What little I did know, I would try to use to my advantage when mouthing off my liberal views during political arguments with friends, coworkers, or family members.

"I think it's a disgrace that poor people in this country have to go without medical care simply because they can't afford it. Why, look at Britain and Canada . . . ," I'd say, and then my voice would trail off, as I knew almost nothing about British and Canadian health services except that they were free.

Once I found myself trapped in the very heart of the National Health Service, however, I was consumed with dread. How good could a hospital really be that provides all its services for free? I wondered. During those early days, I mentioned to several of the doctors that I had health insurance.

"Why didn't you say so earlier?" I hoped they might say. "Let's get you out of this place and into a nice private hospital." Instead they looked embarrassed and told me I shouldn't worry too much about things like that, and that a hospital administrator would be in to see me soon.

I had read that Princess Diana had given birth to her boys in a private hospital, so I knew that one existed in London, and it only made sense that all the very best doctors would be there. I assumed that this private hospital was modern and luxurious and relatively quiet and empty, since the majority of British people, lacking insurance, would be forced to opt for the ridiculously attainable free care that I was receiving. I was sure that the administrators at this private hospital, dazzled by my insurance card, would welcome me with open arms, if I could only figure out how to get there.

Finally, toward the end of my first week in the hospital, I received a visitor. He arrived in the ward after breakfast one morning, and, seeing my name on the chart at the end of my bed, he said, "Mrs. Leary?"

"Yes?"

"Roger Bagley. I'm an administrator with the hospital."

"Oh," I said. "Hi."

Roger Bagley looked around and cleared his throat nervously. Gesturing toward my bedside chair, he said, "May I?"

"Of course."

Mr. Bagley perched on the side of the chair.

"So . . . how are you getting on?"

"Um, okay . . . ," I replied.

"Good. Good. I suppose you've never stayed in a British hospital before . . . ?"

"No."

"Well, I'm sorry you had to experience one under these circumstances, but I hope everything is to your liking."

"Yes, everything's fine," I said. "But I'm not sure if I'm really supposed to be in this particular hospital. I actually have health insurance, and . . ."

"Ah, yes," Mr. Bagley said. He seemed immensely relieved. "Would it be possible for me to contact somebody from your insurance company, then? We just need to certify that . . . well, since you're not a British citizen, and you aren't eligible for free services . . ." Mr. Bagley was clearly embarrassed, as if he had just served me a meal in his home but was now asking me to chip in and pay for it.

"Oh, of course," I said, removing my insurance card from my wallet. "But, since I do have insurance, shouldn't I be at a private hospital?"

"A private hospital?" Mr. Bagley echoed. "No, private hospitals aren't equipped to deal with high-risk pregnancies like yours. Portland Hospital is only a few blocks from here—that's where all the royals and pop stars have their babies. Some of our own doctors have a private practice there as well, but if a mother or baby develops any problems, they're rushed here."

"Oh," I said. "I imagined that the private hospital would be somehow . . . better. Not that this isn't . . . just great. I mean, I love it here, but . . ."

Mr. Bagley smiled. "Don't worry, you're in the right place. We have some of the best doctors in the country here at UCH."

Now I was relieved. Surely some of the best doctors in Britain must be up to par with American doctors, I thought, in my hopelessly American way. Mr. Bagley took my card and examined it.

"So shall I just ring them at this number, then?" he asked.

"Yes," I said. "That's my policy number on the front."

I was touched by Mr. Bagley's discomfort at having to discuss payment with me, and I thought about a time when I had slammed my pinkie in a car door and was allowed to bleed all over a Boston hospital clerk's office while she grilled me on my insurance data.

THE DAYS IN the ward quickly settled into a routine. At seven-thirty breakfast was served. This was always an assortment of rolls and pastries, cornflakes, yogurt, hard-boiled eggs, and some kind of fresh fruit, set up family style on the table in the middle of the room. After breakfast the ward doctor, usually Scott or another young doctor named Dr. Ubin, would do his rounds with one or two resident doctors or medical students. I have to admit that I began to look forward to the doctors' rounds, perhaps a bit too much. In what I can now only believe was some manifestation of the Stockholm syndrome, I had developed crushes on Scott and Dr. Ubin, as well as on Mr. Prosser, my consultant. I found myself blushing when they visited each morning, and when they attempted conversation, I was able to speak only in monosyllables punctuated by guttural, snorting giggles. *Was it my imagination, or did Scott linger after that last examination?* I wondered one morning after he had left. I cursed myself for not asking Denis to bring me some cosmetics, and I passed away many of the long hours fantasizing about being married to a London doctor.

Every morning, the minute the doctors finished their rounds, most of the other women in the ward would file down to the smoking room for a "fag." I can't begin to describe how deeply I resented this. I had quit smoking several months before conceiving my baby and would allow nothing alcoholic or caffeinated to cross my lips. These girls, who smoked like chimneys and moaned about how they wished they could run across the street to the pub for a pint, were going to have big, whopping healthy babies, while my baby would be lucky if it weighed two pounds. The girls grew increasingly friendly toward Denis, and I was annoyed to learn that during his frequent "walks" around the hospital, he was actually in the smoking room with my ward mates. I pictured them all laughing it up, flirting, and bumming cigarettes off each other like high-school kids. These girls, who were still slightly standoffish toward me, apparently shared their life stories with Denis, and he would then fill me in on why they were here in the hospital.

"That's Cindy," he'd say quietly, nodding toward one of my neighbors. "She has genital herpes, so they're going to deliver her by C-section."

"Herpes?" I replied. "She told you that?"

"Well, yeah," Denis said. "I feel sorry for her. She's only nineteen years old."

"Hmmmm," I said.

"What?"

"Did you and the girls have a pillow fight at your little pajama party?"

"What're you talking about?"

"It sounds so cozy down there in that smoking lounge, that's all," I said, and I wondered then who I was. I had never been jealous or catty in my life. I hated women who were, but now, lying swollen, belly-up on large sheets of absorbent disposable bed liners, I felt defective and vulnerable, and the ripe, overdue young girls floating in and out of the ward together, whispering and giggling in their crisp accents and fuzzy slippers, seemed to be somehow mocking me, though they rarely looked my way.

Morning, for me, was the longest part of the day. From the moment breakfast was cleared, I began eyeing the clock to see if it was almost lunchtime. My days had become a series of meals. There was nothing else on the agenda for me, and I began to understand why the animals at the zoo get so restless at feeding time. It's the highlight of their day. Now it was mine. Lunch was served at twelve-thirty, and Denis would usually arrive sometime after that. He always brought me food and magazines, and he usually hung out for the afternoon with me, and we ate the food and looked at all the magazines. Then, as six o'clock approached, he would leave. It was time for tea, and then the long night stretched before me.

I still couldn't read anything more than picture captions. I was filled with anxiety. Crossword puzzles were possible but would take me days, as I had the attention span of a chigger, so I occupied my days and nights alternately crying and spying on my roommates and their visitors. One of the night nurses, a sweet, soft-spoken Irish girl named Claire, told me I should try knitting. She said that the repetitive motion and concentration that knitting requires make it an excellent way to relax. Claire kindly brought me some yarn and some knitting needles the next night. She showed me how to "cast" the row onto the needle, and then she began, effortlessly, to knit. The gentle stabbing of the needles, the clear clacking sound as they met, and the graceful arching patterns performed by the girl's hands had me almost instantly lulled into a contented trance. She knitted a few rows and talked to me about her mother in Belfast, who had taught her to knit as a little girl, and when she stopped, I begged her to continue.

"I need to watch you knit a little more, and then I'll get the hang of it," I said.

She clickety-clacked away, describing her flat in Maida Vale, and her flatmates, and a party they had thrown the night before for a friend who was moving back to Ireland. "There," she said. "Now you have a go."

"More," I begged. "Let me watch you a little more."

"You can do it," she said cheerfully. She handed me the two needles that were now attached to each other by a thin, neatly woven wool panel, and the instant they were in my hands, the needles slipped free and the knitting came unraveled and lay in a tangled heap on my lap.

My attempts at knitting were pathetic and downright dangerous, as one of the needles would occasionally slip from my fingers and shoot like a missile right at my eye. Yarn is slippery, and so are plastic knitting needles, and I thought that when this was all over, I might invent a new knitting needle—short and fat, with a sandpaper finish—and market it for beginning knitters like myself. I hadn't been taught anything new in years, and I realized that whatever capabilities I'd once had for retaining and processing information were now gone. Again and again Claire would explain the simple knot one must tie at the beginning of the line. Then she would show me how to hold the yarn and how to move the needle over, under, and through it. I watched carefully. Then, when it was my turn, I was stumped in the middle of the knot-tying part. I was determined, though, and I tried for days to figure it all out. The idea of hand-knitting the baby's very first sweater was hugely appealing to me, and I imagined him or her delicately lifting it out of a cedar chest one day and unfolding it before the mesmerized eyes of my grandchildren. "Your granny knitted this, bless her soul, while in hospital waiting for me to be born," my child would explain, and the eyes of my grandchildren would mist over with tears of familial love. Ultimately I ended up with a knotted, twisted cord, which I decided would do all right as the baby's first belt.

By the end of my first week in the hospital, all the women who'd been on the ward when I arrived had given birth and gone home, except for Sophie, who had required a cesarean and was recovering in the postnatal ward down the hall. Now there were new patients in the ward, including a Japanese woman who spoke not a word of English and a Nigerian woman, and I felt less like the gate-crasher at a family picnic.

One morning Sophie brought her baby girl, Nicole, in to see me.

"You can hold her if you like," Sophie said. I was very moved that she would allow me to hold her baby, and I reached out my hands for the chubby newborn. She was adorable, like most babies, and as I admired her, Sophie told me about her labor and delivery, and I hung on every word. I couldn't get enough.

"Did you have to beg for the epidural, or did they just give it to you?" I asked. "Could you hear them cutting the skin?" "Could you feel it?" "Did the baby cry the minute she was born?" "Did you hold her?" "Did you nurse her?"

Sophie happily answered all my questions, and then, to my surprise, she asked if I would watch Nicole while she took a shower.

"Won't the nurses take her to the nursery?" I asked.

"What nursery?" asked Sophie.

At UCH, I discovered, the only nursery is the neonatal unit. When a woman has a healthy newborn, the baby is her responsibility, even if she needs to stay on in the hospital to recover from the birth. When the mother has to use the telephone or bathroom, she asks another mother to keep an eye on her baby's "cot," just in case a crazed baby abductor should wander through the ward at exactly that moment.

Our ward was quite chilly at night, and I asked Sophie if they kept the postnatal ward warmer for the babies.

"No," said Sophie, "but they tuck the babies into our beds with us, and they stay warm that way."

I told her that American hospitals, in an effort to avoid expensive lawsuits, had pretty much done away with the practice of allowing babies to be carried around by their mothers, and the thought of allowing a baby to sleep in a bed with a grown woman would be considered lunacy.

Sophie wheeled in her baby's tiny cot, and I felt almost like a normal mom, just watching another mom's baby while she took a shower.

An Orthodox Jewish woman was admitted to the ward over the weekend. Her husband was with her, as was an older woman who appeared to be the pregnant woman's mother. I noticed that I wasn't the only other patient who stole glances at the family, not only because of the women's wigs and the man's black suit but also because they were all speaking on cell phones. It's hard to imagine now, only thirteen years later, that a time existed when a person carrying a telephone around in a pocket was a source of fascination. Later that evening, when visiting hours were over, the Orthodox woman removed her wig, then touched her belly, as we all did when our babies moved, and I felt instantly that she had more in common with us than with the family who had brought her. I thought of a documentary I'd once seen about a primitive tribe in South America or Africa. In this tribe women leave their families before they give birth and stay in a birthing hut, where no men are allowed. They remain in the hut with other expectant mothers until, a month later, they emerge with their babies. During the evenings, after the men had left, the antenatal ward felt a little like a birthing hut. In the middle of the night, I would awaken to hear one of my roommates turning restlessly in bed, her labor beginning. A sister would arrive with a fetal monitor and strap it around the woman's belly, and I would listen to the sounds of her baby's heart beating, many fathoms deep. Sometimes more than one monitor would be going, the dueling heart sounds rising and falling. I would touch my belly, my baby would roll leisurely against my hand, and it was hard to imagine then that a world existed outside that room.

I WAS ABLE to fall asleep each night when the lights were lowered in the ward, but I usually awoke with a start several hours later. A shaft of gray light from the hall always shone through the center of the room, illuminating only the bottom half of each bed, and from the mysterious region beyond the ward could be heard the sounds of urgent footsteps on hard tiled floors. Though the nights were cold and damp, the windows were usually cracked open. From the streets below rose the sounds of a foreign city—distant sirens and the occasional diluted hollering of a drunk—and it always took me a few moments to recall that I was in a London maternity hospital. Then, once again, my self-interrogation would begin. Why did I get on that plane? Did I lift something too heavy? Why hadn't I stayed home and rested, instead of trotting halfway across the globe, jeopardizing my poor baby's life? Sometimes a pair of nurses would enter the room and stand whispering at the foot of one of the beds, and I would close my eyes and force myself to breathe slowly and feign sleep.

From the moment I was admitted to UCH, I was filled with remorse and fear and dread, but I desperately tried to hide it from the attending nurses and physicians. I knew that the British expected a stiff upper lip in situations like this, and I knew it because of a favorite piece of reading material that I'd cherished as a young teen.

I found the manual while baby-sitting for the Gardner children. Ever since I had discovered Anaïs Nin's *Delta of Venus* at another baby-sitting job, I made it a habit to inspect all employers' bookshelves after the children had gone to bed. The Gardners' bookshelves were initially a big disappointment. There was no erotic literature, only a few volumes of Reader's Digest condensed novels, a series of Time-Life books on home repair, some hunting guides, and a thick pamphlet that, when I pulled it off the shelf, I discovered was a poorly photocopied military manual that had been written by senior officers of the Royal Air Force, and its purpose was to teach younger enlisted men survival techniques. I'm not sure how Mr. Gardner had obtained this pamphlet, but he was a gun aficionado and a Vietnam vet, and I have a feeling that his wife and kids have since left him and he is at this very moment holed up in a cabin in Montana, awaiting an armed standoff with the Bureau of Alcohol, Tobacco and Firearms.

Anyway, I read this pamphlet from cover to cover. I read it again each time I baby-sat. I read it with the same degree of fascination and horror with which I had read *Delta of Venus,* and I fantasized about someday finding myself in a life-or-death situation where I might have to use some of the techniques I had learned in this incredible manual, hopefully with a British air force officer at my side.

The manual was divided into chapters that covered the most common military survival situations. One chapter was devoted to surviving enemy prison camps, while others discussed survival at sea, in hostile enemy territory, and in the desert. These chapters contained many anecdotes about the actual wartime experiences of the authors, and each one commanded a pull-yourself-up-by-the-bootstraps mentality that spoke volumes about the resourcefulness (and lack of tolerance for whiners) of the British.

The prison-camp chapter was my favorite. I was raised on daily doses of *Hogan's Heroes,* and *The Great Escape* is one of my favorite movies. For me, the wartime prison camp ranked just below the western cattle ranch in favorite fantasy destinations, and when you're in junior high school, you need someplace to go during Algebra 1. Sure, the accommodations aren't luxurious, but the adrenaline-pumping danger combined with the built-in romantic possibilities gave me endless material to occupy my mind throughout most of my school day.

According to the manual's prison-camp chapter, the most important thing a POW must do is eat. The problem is that the food is usually so rancid that flies and maggots are already eating it. The authors explain that the fatal error committed by many is to refuse the food. The food must be eaten, maggots and all. Maggots, it turns out, are an excellent source of protein. Not only that, the best thing for a fresh wound, lacking iodine or sutures, is the maggot, who will eat only the dead and decaying flesh and thereby help prevent infection. I think you're starting to get the picture here.

My favorite character—in my opinion the hero of the manual—was the British officer in the chapter about survival tools. This chapter was devoted almost entirely to the knife. Leaving your knife at home, according to RAF officers, is tantamount to swallowing cyanide. A knife can be fastened to a branch and used as a spear to hunt food. It can cut a bullet out of your thigh or slit the throat of your captor. In fact, one of the authors asked the reader what a colleague of his would have done without his knife when he stepped on a land mine in France. Not only did this man use his knife to amputate his leg, but he was then able to whittle a crutch from a tree limb and make his way back to his unit.

It was compelling reading, impossible to put down, and now that I found myself imprisoned in a foreign hospital, I took solace in recalling the mettle of those British soldiers and was determined that nobody find out what a wuss I really was.

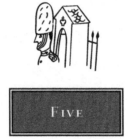

FIVE

M Y MOTHER'S HUSBAND, Stephen Howe, is a devoted Anglophile, and the year they married, he took my mother on her first trip to England. Although they were there for only a week she returned with a slight British accent and an alarmingly transformed vocabulary. Pants had become trousers. My mother now rode the lift, not the elevator. Her car ran on petrol, and when she needed the loo—say, at the cinema—she would sometimes have to queue up. "Is this the queue?" she would ask the others in line at the local multiplex, and they would shrug and shake their heads in confusion. My sister, Meg, and I teased her about this mercilessly.

"'Ow about a nice cuppa tea, Mum," I'd say when she told

us that she and Steve had "hired" a video the night before.

"Blimey!" Meg would say. "It's teatime already, is it? I'll get the jam from the cupboard."

"Is the guv'nor about?" I'd ask. "I'd like to say 'ello to old Steve. Then I'm off to the pub with me mates."

"I fancy a nice pint meself," Meg would say, and we would carry on like that until one of us had wet our trousers. Meg and I consider ourselves screamingly funny and can whip each other into a state of crying, peeing hysteria in a matter of minutes. My mother would insist that she had no idea what we were talking about. "I've always said 'hire,'" she'd insist. "That's not a British word."

Every year after that first trip, my mother and Steve returned to England in June to visit their friends the Thwaites, who live in Henley-on-Thames. Each year they attended the races at Royal Ascot and sat in a special box situated quite close to the queen herself. My mother had been all over London. She'd been to Harrods and to Covent Garden. She knew her way across Hyde Park to Buckingham Palace, where she had viewed the changing of the guard. She had visited the Houses of Parliament and the Tower of London. It would be very easy for her to come and be with me, she said to me now, as I lay in a maternity ward in Central London. She said that London was like a second home to her, but I suspected that the London my mother knew was slightly different from the London where I now resided.

* * *

I WAS AWARE of my mother's arrival at UCH long before I laid eyes on her. Nobody wears high heels in hospitals, but, given the opportunity, my mother would wear high heels on a hike across the Sahara. I heard the familiar strike of her heels as she approached. I heard them growing louder, coming nearer, and suddenly there she was.

Now that I have children of my own, I know that it's normal for them to go through a stage when they're embarrassed by their parents. My kids are firmly entrenched in this stage now, and although I'm told they'll grow out of it, I have my doubts, because *I* never did. If it had been somebody else's mother who arrived that afternoon dressed in a tailored blue suit, sporting a jaunty hat, and laden with Harrods bags, I would have thought her charming. But this was *my* mother, and in my mind she'd just arrived in the ward wearing nothing but a neon placard with the word "Yankee" emblazoned upon it. Again, regressing to about the fifth grade, I thought simultaneously, *Thank God, Mom's here* and *I hope nobody figures out she's my mom.*

"HI, ANNIE!" she called from the door. I gave her a feeble wave. She clicked her way across the floor and waved and said hello to the other women in their beds, who were trying not to stare. When she reached my bedside, she gave me one of her careful, tentative hugs, then sat down on a chair beside me.

"I WOULD HAVE COME EARLIER, BUT I WANTED

TO STOP AND GET YOU A FEW THINGS, DARLING.
HOW ARE YOU FEELING?" she said, and as she continued
with questions about my condition and the baby's, I wondered
if she had always spoken this loudly. How was it possible that
she had learned all those British words but had not picked up
on the fact that British people speak very quietly in public?

"Mom," I whispered, "we're supposed to keep our voices
down. There are babies sleeping in some of the other rooms."

"Was I being loud?" my mother asked. Then she said, "I
spoke to Joan Thwaites. She says this is an excellent hospital."

"I know," I said.

"She said you'd be crazy to GO TO A PRIVATE HOSPI-
TAL—"

"Shhhh!" I hissed.

"What?" my mother said.

"I don't know, maybe your ears are filled from the flight over.
You're talking really loudly," I said, and immediately I hated
myself for caring what the others thought. I have always been
my mother's worst critic. When I was a child, living in Michigan
and Wisconsin, all my friends were envious of my mother.
"She's so cool and pretty," they'd say. Or "I wish my mom could
wear hot pants." These girls had mothers whose thighs required
polyester stretch pants. Moms who frosted their own hair,
served Hamburger Helper for dinner, and in the evenings
watched *Hee Haw* with Dad.

My mom was slender and stylish and clever. She would
admire a caftan worn by Lauren Hutton in *Vogue* and sew one

up for herself that very day. She had the ability to walk into a Piggly Wiggly supermarket in Kenosha, Wisconsin, and walk out with the ingredients for moules au beurre d'escargots, which she would prepare that evening for dinner, just for the family. She read Russian history, hated midwestern accents, smoked More cigarettes (the long, thin brown ones that look like effeminate cigars), and absolutely loved a good party. All my childhood friends were mortified by their own mothers, and they thought mine was the best, but at times, as a child, I secretly coveted theirs—the mothers with doughy arms, twinkly smiles, and arsenals of homespun wisdom such as "The proof is in the pudding" and "Pretty is as pretty does."

On her second day in London, my mother arrived at my bedside with the *International Herald Tribune*. She pulled her chair up close to my bed and, opening the paper, showed me the *New York Times* crossword puzzle. I was seized with panic.

My mother does the *Times* crossword puzzle every day. On Mondays she can do the puzzle in ten minutes while talking on the phone. As the week progresses and the puzzle becomes more challenging, it takes up more of her day, and by Saturday she sits surrounded by dictionaries and encyclopedias and solves the puzzle with the single-minded determination of a scientist unraveling the mysteries of DNA. On weekdays there's nobody around to admire her acuity with the English language, so on Sundays, when her husband and, often, one or more of her children are present, she tries to turn what should be a solitary diversion into a one-woman performance piece designed to showcase her superior intellect.

She usually waits until we're all seated in the family room reading the Sunday papers, and then she innocently settles herself into her favorite armchair. She works quietly for a few moments, then sighs and says, to no one in particular, "I'm having the hardest time with today's puzzle." In response we all shake our papers and squint fiercely at the pages, trying to convey the seriousness of our reading and the imperviousness of our concentration. This is lost on my mother, who then scans the room looking for her first victim.

"Denis," she said one Sunday years ago, when Denis was still concerned with making a good impression, "you'll know this. . . . I need a Revolutionary War general."

Denis, naïve to the tyranny of the puzzler, good-naturedly tried to get in the spirit of things.

"George Washington!" he announced proudly.

"No," my mother said. "There are only four letters."

"I'm sure you'll figure it out, Mom," I said, trying to rescue Denis.

"C'mon," my mother said. "You should know this, Annie. Steve . . . darling . . . a Revolutionary War general?"

Steve looked up from his paper and, frowning, said the first thing that came to his mind:

"Paul Revere."

Then he looked back at his paper.

My mother tried to suppress her laughter. "Are you serious?" she asked.

Steve continued with his reading.

"Darling," she said, "you must be joking. Paul Revere was a member of the militia and not a general." Then she looked at us and rolled her eyes, sighing.

Steve is an attorney and, thus challenged, was compelled to defend himself.

"Of course Paul Revere was a militiaman. You don't think the militia had ranks, had officers?" Steve said this sternly, in the hopes that it would dissuade my mother from pursuing her line of questioning, but he should have known better, as she responded, "Well, I'm certainly aware that the militia had ranks, but they didn't have generals or colonels, per se—isn't that right, Denis?"

"Ummm . . . ," Denis said. "What are the other letters?"

"Well, that's the problem," my mother said. "I have the first letter as G. I know that's right, because it's from eight down— Giza, which is a Cairo suburb. So of course I thought Gage, as in Thomas Gage, the famous British general. The problem is, if it's Gage, the A doesn't work . . . wait a minute, I was looking at the wrong clue for twenty-six down. 'Lethargic feeling' is the clue. That would be 'malaise,' right, Annie?"

"What?" I said, looking up from my paper.

"'Malaise.' That works. Okay, Steve, here's one you'll love: 'Stow on a boat.'"

Steve was now forced to feign deafness. He moved his paper closer to his face and frowned thoughtfully at his news.

"Steve."

"Hmmm?"

"'Stow on a boat.'"

"I think the word is 'stow.'"

"'Steeve.' The word is 'steeve.' With two *es*. You really should have known that, Steve!" my mother said, laughing. "Now we're getting someplace. Annie, here's one for you: 'Monkey Trial locale,' six letters."

"Africa," I said.

"Oh, for heaven's sake, Annie. The Scopes Monkey Trial?"

"Darrow!" Denis announced triumphantly. "Darrow, Tennessee."

"Oh, that's right!" I said, thinking, *Take that! My boyfriend's not as dumb as he looks.*

"Darrow, Tennessee! Too funny!" my mother exclaimed. "Clarence Darrow was the lawyer for the evolutionist on trial! The trial was in Dayton, Tennessee! This is great fun, isn't it?"

And so she continued throughout the day, until the puzzle was done and the entire family was suitably demoralized by the fresh evidence of our staggering stupidity.

Denis is fiercely competitive and grew to resent the puzzle more than the rest of us did. "You know," he said to her once, when she'd asked him to name a San Joaquin Valley city, "if I liked crossword puzzles, I'd do them myself." To which my mother replied, "Crossword puzzles are meant to be done as a group!"

"But we're *not* doing it as a group," Denis said. "You've already answered the easy ones, and now you're tormenting everybody with the ones nobody knows."

"Here's one you'll know: Who was Superman's mother? Four letters. C'mon, this is the last one I'll ask."

So I sat in my metal hospital bed and participated in the puzzling. I couldn't figure out a way of explaining how annoying it was without hurting her feelings. I've never been able to confront my mother about certain tendencies she has, because, according to a therapist I started going to later, I suffer from fears of abandonment. "Doesn't everybody?" I asked her. "Who wants to be abandoned?"

My mother doesn't believe in therapy, which is a shame, not because I think she would benefit in any way from it but because her childhood was a veritable treasure trove of dysfunction, and it lies fallow, purposely locked away in her mind. I think it's a crime that analysts sit listening to people like me whine about this slight or that misunderstanding when somebody like my mother walks about with rich secrets buried beneath the perky mantle of modified reality she has created. It's like somebody with a collection of rare first-edition books stored away in a damp, moldy basement, unaware of its worth to collectors and curators.

Whenever I ask my mother about her childhood, she sighs heavily and acts as if I've just asked her to conjugate verbs in Latin. It's all too tedious for words, is the impression she likes to give, but the tidbits I've wrenched from her in moments of weakness or drunkenness are astonishingly sad. Her father, Eugene, went off to fight in World War II and never returned. He returned from the war, but not to her home, and her mother, abandoned and bitter, moved my mother and her brother from Philadelphia to rural northern Pennsylvania, where my grandmother could thoroughly indulge her alcoholism and depression. My mother was a lonely child who couldn't bring friends home from school for fear they would find my grandmother "out of sorts."

Once, when my grandmother had suffered some form of collapse, my grandfather came to get the kids. My grandfather was a salesman in New York, living in a single room, so he dropped my mom and her brother at the home of a friend who had a wife and children. My mother, who was apparently about seven years old and had never met these people before, cried inconsolably for a day or two. When Eugene came to get my mother, he had some harsh words for her in the car. This caused her to cry again, whereupon he turned around and ordered her to stop. And I imagine that there was something in his tone or demeanor that was terrifying, because my mother did stop crying, and to this day she is proud to be able to say that she's not an emotional person.

Denis's mother, Nora, on the other hand, is happy to tell stories about her childhood, and who wouldn't be, with a childhood as quaint and picturesque as hers? There were six siblings in her family's home, which was on a dairy farm, and their house had no electricity or running water. Each day the milk was hauled to the village in the back of a pony cart. A large stone fireplace heated the entire house, fueled with sod that the men and children carved out of nearby bogs. The children walked three miles to school each morning and then three miles home in the afternoons. In the evenings, for entertainment, the family sat around kerosene lanterns and told stories, or somebody would play the fiddle, or a child would dance.

Each spring Nora's father sprinkled holy water, blessed by the parish priest, on his fields as a blessing for the new season's crops. One year, when Nora was quite small, she and one of her sisters were sent to Killarney to fetch a bucket of holy water from the church. It was a long walk from their farm to Killarney, and Nora and her sister began fooling around a little bit on the way home. Eventually Nora started swinging the bucket of holy water over her head and was marveling at the powers of centrifugal force when the handle broke. The holy water spilled all over the road and trickled down into a ditch. Nora and her sister were terrified. A spanking was in store for them, they knew, if they showed up at home with an empty bucket, so they filled the bucket with water from a nearby stream. That evening the family said a prayer and Nora's father took a branch from an evergreen and dipped it into the bucket of water. Then he sprinkled the stream water all over his newly seeded fields. Nora spent many sleepless nights worrying about the day when the seeds would sprout, rotted with blight, reeking and fermented. "But," said Nora, "wouldn't you know the beans and potatoes came in that year bigger and healthier than any year before or since!"

The day Denis's younger sister was born, their father, John, wanted to buy Nora flowers, but payday wasn't until the next day, and he had no money. As he walked to the hospital, a five-dollar bill flew across the street and plastered itself against his pant leg. This is a favorite Leary story, as it summarizes how things often turn out for them, luck and birth and family all happily intertwined.

PART TWO

Special Care

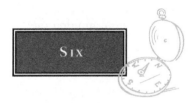

*I*N THE UNITED States, neonatal units are referred to by the clinical-sounding term "Neonatal Intensive Care Unit," or NICU (pronounced *NICK-you*). In Britain they are given a cuddlier name—"Special Care Baby Unit," or SCBU (pronounced SKI-boo). One day, when my mother was visiting, a sister named Chris came to see me. She was from the SCBU and brought a photo album filled with pictures of premature babies. She said that the neonatal staff, when possible, thought it was helpful to prepare parents for what their baby would look like and what life was like in the SCBU.

I opened the photo album. I had seen preemies on news programs, and the babies in these photos were of the same breed. They were almost indistinguishable from one another, with their pinched faces and tube-filled noses, their splayed poses seemingly inspired by science-lab frogs. Each infant's date of birth and gestational age were printed underneath its photo. In some cases there was a picture of a fat, healthy, finished-looking baby next to the preemie, with a later date printed underneath. "Is that the same baby?" I asked, hopefully, and Chris said, "Yes!" and then she showed me some more before-and-after photos. Most of the after photos revealed perfectly normal-looking babies, and when I commented enthusiastically about this, Chris said that most babies who leave the unit *are* normal in the long run, but she reminded me that many of the babies are only a few weeks premature when they're born. Chris then offered to take us downstairs for a tour of the unit, and my mother and I accepted gratefully.

From the third-floor ward, we took an elevator down to a narrow corridor that led right into the SCBU. There were four separate rooms in the SCBU, Chris told us, and we began by looking in Room D, which was the room for babies who are almost ready to go home. These babies were either born recently, only slightly premature, or had been born several months before and had graduated to Room D, after making their way through Rooms A, B, and C. In Room C, there were four other relatively healthy babies, all in the three-to-four-pound range. Rooms A and B held smaller, sicker babies, and although I had seen photographs, I was overwhelmed by the sight of these tiny infants.

Very-low-birth-weight premature babies have straight limbs. This, to me, more than their tiny size or wizened facial features, is what causes them to appear most unbabylike. A full-term baby spends its final few months tightly hugged by the womb and is born with knees and elbows folded, a chubby package designed to fit perfectly in the crook of an arm. Preemies lie flat, like marionettes before a show, their legs and arms straight, skin draped across bone. The heat in the isolette makes their skin dry, and Chris told us that their lips must be dabbed constantly with Vaseline to keep them from cracking. These tiny babies didn't cry—they just slept—but I sensed their awful solitude. I imagined that if they had any consciousness or sensibility at all, it would be that life now was hard, and it had once been warm, fluid, and easy.

Chris showed us a baby who'd been born at twenty-seven weeks' gestation, which was about my baby's gestational age. He was lying on a flat table, and Chris explained that when premature infants are first born, they're placed on these warming beds, which are basically just heated tables. This helps the infants stay warm and also allows the doctors and nurses easy access to them. Once their body temperature becomes stable, they're moved into an isolette—the covered incubator with two holes on the side for caregivers' arms. As we gazed at this baby, his grandparents arrived to have a first look at their grandson. They stared at him silently, and then, as we turned to leave, I heard the grandfather say quietly to his wife, "The poor little mite."

Chris wheeled me back to the elevator. The ride up to the ward was silent. She told me that if I had any questions at any time I could send for her. When she left, my mother said, "That was so nice of her, wasn't it?" and I burst into tears. My mother turned away from me then, and I saw that she was crying, too, my mother who never cries.

WHEN I WAS very young, we lived in Maryland in an old house near the Chesapeake Bay. On Saturdays my father used to take my brother and me out rowing on the bay in our dinghy. We would tie a fish head to a piece of string and lower it into the water. When we pulled it up, there would be a crab, or sometimes two or three, attached to the fish, and my dad would scoop it up in a net for my mom to cook when we got home.

One Saturday my mother, father, brother, sister, and I all crowded into the dinghy, and my father rowed us out to a little island for a picnic. My brother and I explored a nearby pine grove while our parents and baby Meg stayed on the beach. In the shadows of a winding path, partially hidden by a fern, I found a baby bird that had fallen out of its nest. I didn't know what it was at first. It was almost all head. Its legs were curled beneath the mottled gray body, and its wings were just tiny buds. I had never seen anything so naked and frail. Looking closer, I saw that it had a tiny beak and that its eyes, which bulged from the side of its head, were covered by thin, filmy eyelids. The bird opened its beak wide, then closed it, and I carefully picked it up. I was amazed at its weightlessness. I cradled the bird in my hand. When I held it up in front of my face, its moist head drooped against my thumb.

Carefully, tenderly, I carried the hatchling down to the beach in my hands, but when I showed it to my parents, my mother smiled sadly and said, "You shouldn't have touched it."

"Why not?" I asked.

"Because now the mother won't want to take care of it."

We all walked back to the place where I had found it, and we looked in the trees above for a nest, but there wasn't one.

"You have to leave it here," my mother said.

"But it'll die," I protested.

"It'll die anyway," my mother said. "Leave it alone."

I held the bird against my face and felt the soft pulse of its heart against my palm. I started crying. When my mother tried to get the bird away from me, I became hysterical. Finally she relented angrily, shaking her head and stomping back to the dinghy. I pulled up the bottom of my T-shirt and made a little hammock for the bird, then climbed into the boat.

On the way home, I held my hand over the small, warm lump in my shirt and thought about my bird and our future together. I would name him Sweetie and feed him from an eyedropper. When he grew, I would walk around the neighborhood with him on my shoulder, and all the neighborhood kids would run out to the sidewalk to watch us pass. I would teach Sweetie to fly, and the day would come when I would set him free, only to have him circle back to me after one glorious soar above the neighborhood. Sweetie would live the rest of his life as my half-wild bird friend. When I left school each afternoon, he would swoop down from the tree where he'd spent the entire day watching me through my classroom window. I would walk home with Sweetie flying just above my head, and the other kids would point to me and shout, "There she is! There's the girl who tames birds!" and they would crowd around me murmuring in awe, begging to be my friend. As my father rowed us back to the mainland, these thoughts built to a crescendo of ecstatic delusion. Catching my mother's eye, I smiled with delight. She mistook the smile for a gloating smirk related to her defeat in our battle of wills, and she said, also smiling but staring fixedly into my eyes, "You are a spoiled brat."

That night I tried to feed the bird from an eyedropper filled with milk, but the milk dribbled out the sides of its beak. I dug up a worm and tried to place it in the baby's beak, as a mother bird might, but the baby didn't seem to know what to do with it. I tried to ignore the stabbing pangs of guilt I felt when I recalled my mother's words about how I shouldn't have touched the baby bird in the first place. If I had left it on the island, would the mother bird be feeding it now? I imagined the baby nestling down with its mother for the night, its nude, unfinished form tucked safely beneath her warm, feathered breast.

My mother helped me fill a shoe box with grass and leaves, to keep the bird warm, and we put the box high on a shelf where our cat couldn't get it. The next morning I woke my dad up early and begged him to get the box down for me. I waited expectantly as he carefully lowered the box. Surely the bird would be stronger today, I thought. Maybe its eyes would be open. Maybe it would recognize my scent and understand that I was its new mother. But it had died in the night, and my father buried it beneath a bush in our backyard. "It's better to leave them alone," my father said as he carried the box outside.

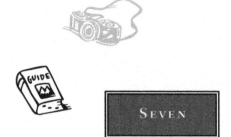

SEVEN

URING OUR SECOND week in London, Denis visited with me during the day, and during the evenings he made his B and B money performing at the Comedy Store and various other clubs in and around London. It's hard to imagine now how Denis managed to perform onstage and be funny during such a crisis, but he'd been doing stand-up for years. It was his only source of income. Often one gig would be our entire rent. He got onstage when he was sick, when he was tired, even the night several years earlier when his beloved father had died.

He'd never had such a succession of knockout performances as the one he was experiencing in London, however. It seemed that the British audiences loved Denis's edgier material, so he came up with some new stuff, and they loved that, too. The producers of the Paramount City show booked Denis for a repeat performance on the Saturday after his original show, and we were very grateful for their generosity.

The day of that second Paramount City performance turned out to be one that would find itself on the pages of Britain's history books. It was March 31, 1990, the day of the infamous poll-tax riots in London. Until that March I had lived my entire life happily unaware of anything associated with British politics and national affairs. I knew that the prime minister was Margaret Thatcher, that she was a Conservative crony of Reagan and Bush, and . . . well, that was about it. How was I to know that Thatcher was devising an overhaul of the nation's system of taxation in a manner so unfair and illogical that thousands of people would take to the streets in a demonstration that would turn violent and cause my husband and Dire Straits' Mark Knopfler to stand trembling in the vestibule of the Paramount City Theatre, watching their driver's car be set afire? When Denis arrived at the hospital that evening, hours after he'd said he would come visit me, I listened with skepticism to his tales of walking through rioting crowds.

"Really, all you have to say is that you wanted to hang out with Mark Knopfler," I said to him.

"Honey, I'm telling you, there were people turning over parked cars. I saw a mounted cop take out a guy with his bat, right in front of me!"

"Right, right, whatever," I said. "Please lower your voice. There's no reason everybody in this room has to hear your convoluted excuses."

*   *   *

I MET DENIS at Emerson College in Boston, in the fall of 1982. The summer before, I'd been planning to return for my third year at Bennington College in Vermont, when I awoke one morning with the urgent realization that I couldn't bear another Vermont winter. I wanted to be in a city. I applied to Emerson's Department of Creative Writing and Literature just a few weeks before school was scheduled to begin in the fall, and, amazingly, I was accepted.

The head of the writing department, Dr. James Randall, had encouraged me to sign up for a class called Comedy Writing. Dr. Randall explained that Norman Lear, an Emerson alumnus, sent a representative to review material from the class each winter and had hired a few writers for his television shows over the years. The girl who was hired the year before was now living in Los Angeles and earning an astounding $700 a week. At the time I was earning $120 a week working in a flower shop on Charles Street. Seven hundred dollars every week seemed like a scandalously exorbitant amount of money. What would a person do with all that money? I wondered greedily. I hastily signed up for the class and left Dr. Randall's office dizzy with hope and longing. *I'm funny,* I thought. *All my friends tell me I'm funny.* I walked down Beacon Street and envisioned myself sitting around a table with my classmates. I watched them read my material and convulse with laughter, pounding their desks with their fists and gasping for breath, tears streaming down their faces. I imagined the flight to Los Angeles, accompanied by the scout who refused to leave me in Boston another minute. Then I saw myself at a table surrounded by staff writers, who were writhing in their seats, screaming with laughter at my script suggestions. The Mercedes convertible, the house in Malibu, the closet filled with Italian shoes—it was all suddenly within my grasp thanks to Dr. Randall's suggestion that I take a class taught by a comedy writer named Mr. Leary.

On the first day of the comedy class, nine other students and I sat in a classroom when a young man walked in and leaned on the desk in the front of the room. At first I assumed that the skinny blond guy was another student, but he greeted us in a welcoming sort of way, and then he sat on the desk. The teacher's desk. This couldn't possibly be Mr. Denis Leary, the teacher on my registration form, I thought. It occurred to me that he might have been the student assistant/gay lover of the teacher (I had just transferred from Bennington) and was filling in while Mr. Leary screened calls from Hollywood agents desperate for writers.

"Hi, I'm Denis," the man said. Then, lighting a cigarette, he said, "Smoke 'em if you got 'em," and all ten of us pulled out cigarettes and lit up.

The class was fun and the only class I never missed. I had a crush on Denis from the start, and later I learned that everybody else in the class did as well. We wrote short essays that were supposed to be humorous and sample scripts for shows like *Cheers* and *M*A*S*H*. It was the only writing workshop I'd ever participated in where all the members were genuinely kind and supportive of one another. We would always summon up a few chuckles for even the most vapid material and insist that we liked everything that was read, offering only constructive criticism. It was during this class that I came to the sad realization that it's one thing to yuck it up with your friends but another thing altogether to write smart, funny dialogue for television. I was the worst, producing the most hopelessly derivative material, which, my classmates gently had to remind me, had been subconsciously lifted from old *Mary Tyler Moore* and *Gilligan's Island* episodes.

I knew that Denis was attracted to me. He flirted with me in class, but the most obvious giveaway was his habit of wandering casually by the shop where I worked and then, seeing me carrying in containers of flowers from the sidewalk, exclaiming, "You work here? Oh, that's right. I remember you told me." He did this at least twice a week. One time he strode into the store to tell me that a guest speaker from some television studio was coming in the next day. "I know," I replied. "You told us in class." Finally the semester was over. I received one of the only A's in my life, and Denis asked me out on a date. Within two weeks we were living together.

BEFORE GOING TO London, we had lived in a rental apartment in Boston, but Denis also shared a studio in Greenwich

Village with two other comics. He taught his class at Emerson only one more year after we met, and then he did stand-up full-time. He performed in and around Boston regularly, and then he would take the train to New York a few times a month to perform in clubs like Caroline's and Catch A Rising Star in the hopes that he would be discovered by a network scout or Hollywood agent.

In the five years between the time I finished college and became pregnant with Jack, I dabbled in many fields—primarily the waitressing field. I had also worked as a secretary at a real-estate development company, as a casting assistant at a talent agency, and as a copywriter/gofer at a small ad agency. I worked for a while in an archaeology lab and then in a substance-abuse counseling office. I worked as a cashier in one bookstore and then another, but it was difficult holding a day job, fantasizing about becoming a famous novelist, and going out to clubs to watch Denis and our friends perform each night. Early on in our relationship, I thought I had found the perfect solution when the manager of a downtown comedy club asked me if I would work the door a few nights a week. My job was to take the cover charge from customers as they came into the club and then to keep an eye on the audience during the show. If a drunken college kid got loud and disruptive, I was to alert a bouncer and have him removed.

I imagined that I would have plenty of time to write notes for my novel or, if I ever came up with an idea for a plot, to write the actual novel while seated at the back of this club. The nights I worked were usually open-mike nights. These were nights when aspiring comedians would get onstage and do ten minutes of comedy before an audience, sometimes for the very first time. It was during these open-mike nights that I became aware of the sad, demented, insidiously warped mind of the aspiring comedian.

On my first night at work, once everybody had paid and was seated, I sat on a little chair inside the door and watched the opening acts. First an experienced comic, the emcee, did about ten minutes of solid material, and then he would call up the new guys. Some were funnier than others, but toward the middle of the show that first night, an older man was called onto the stage. This man was about forty, and when he took the microphone off the stand, he shook so hard that he caused the amplifier to hum with feedback. His voice trembled when he spoke, and it was clear that the adrenaline rush of walking to the stage in front of all those people had drained his mouth of saliva. His lips stuck together each time he closed his mouth, and swallowing was obviously a very deliberate effort. In this man the audience and I immediately recognized the unbridled fear of the doomed, and I for one wished he would run from the stage and seek the anonymity of the night. But instead he croaked his way through painfully unfunny material, and when a heckler told him to get off the stage, he lost his place and turned beet red and looked like he might cry. He finally finished his act, however, and as he walked from the stage accompanied by a polite smattering of applause, my heart ached with pity.

That's that, I thought. *He'll go back to work tomorrow at his accounting firm and give up this comedian dream for good.* Imagine my shock when he walked up to Craig, the club manager, who was standing a few feet from me.

"What'd you think?" asked the unfunny man.

"Hmmmm? Oh. Well, not too bad," said Craig, without turning his face away from the stage.

"It went good, huh?" said the unfunny man enthusiastically.

"I don't know about 'good,'" replied Craig.

"So how about next Tuesday? Can I go on again?"

"You know . . . I don't think it's a great idea. You need to work on some new stuff. Come back in a month."

"A month then!" said the unfunny man, and he left the club grinning from ear to ear.

Later I learned from Craig that the unfunny guy was an open-mike veteran, that he had some sort of masochistic desire to perform, and that guys like him were a dime a dozen in the comedy world.

When I learned I was pregnant, my stepfather was kind enough to hire me to work at his law firm as a receptionist, so that I could be on an insurance plan. Denis and I lived hand to mouth, earning just enough each month to cover our expenses, and now that we were in London and weren't working, we were rapidly running out of money. But we had a plan.

Denis had an upcoming college gig that would net him enough to cover the rent on both the Boston apartment and the Greenwich Village share. We decided that after the coming weekend, Denis should exchange his first-class return ticket for a round-trip economy ticket and go back to Boston for the college show, which was on a Wednesday night. He could pay our bills and return to London on Thursday. What were the odds that the baby, after waiting all this time, would arrive on one of the few days that Denis would be gone? Both Dr. Ubin and Scott said that he could safely go. The baby had waited this long; it was unlikely to be born anytime soon. It seemed like an excellent plan, and when you're in a hospital, especially a British hospital run by ward matrons and formally attired consultants, it seems possible that even an unborn baby can be persuaded to stick to a plan.

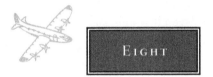

EIGHT

*D*ENIS FLEW FROM Heathrow to JFK on Sunday. When he arrived at the apartment, there was a message on the machine from me. I was going to have the baby within a few hours, was the message. So Denis went back to JFK, and by the time he got to Heathrow the next morning, he had missed not only the college booking but also the birth of his son.

There's really not much to tell about the actual birth. Early Monday morning I awoke feeling some very slight pangs in my lower abdomen. An ultrasound was performed, and it was discovered that the baby was a boy, he was breech, and he was succeeding in working his feet through the birth canal. Mr. Prosser was summoned, and when he arrived, I was rushed into the operating theater for an emergency cesarean.

Obviously it wasn't like the fantasy births I had imagined. For one thing, it was a cesarean, and, for another, my mother was there instead of Denis or a handsome fireman. Mr. Prosser had several residents in attendance, and he explained everything to me before they began. Mine was a complicated delivery and a valuable learning opportunity for the attendants. Since the baby was breech and was surrounded by very little amniotic fluid, instead of the horizontal incision that is usually made on the uterus, Mr. Prosser would perform a classical cesarean—meaning a vertical incision—which would make it easier to retrieve the tiny baby but also meant, Mr. Prosser told me gravely, that I would be able to have only cesareans in future deliveries. In the broad scheme of things, this seemed trivial. That whole vaginal-birth business is overrated, I thought. Let somebody else have a slimy baby plopped onto her belly. There are more important things.

During my time in the antenatal ward, many conversations I had with the other patients inevitably revolved around child-birth, and every imaginable horror story had been divulged. Somebody's sister had had her uterus rupture while pushing out the baby. Another knew a girl whose baby was born dead after thirty-six hours of labor. But the story that haunted me for days was the one about the woman who'd been given an epidural for a cesarean. This woman, somebody's sister's friend, had a rare resistance to the epidural medication. It wasn't until the doctor started cutting that they all realized the epidural hadn't worked and the woman had complete sensation, but they'd already begun the surgery and had to finish cutting the woman open unanesthetized.

When I was all laid out on the operating table and a curtain was hung across my chest so that I couldn't see the gore below, I admit I panicked.

"Wait!" I said. "Wait. I don't think the epidural has taken effect."

"Don't worry," said Mr. Prosser.

"DON'T CUT!" I cried.

"Too late," said Prosser. "We're already inside."

Apparently the epidural had worked after all.

For the benefit of the residents, Mr. Prosser was explaining what he was doing, but he wanted to spare me the details, so he spoke in a cryptic series of half sentences, which I desperately tried to follow.

"There we are. See that . . . ? That's why we have to . . ." Then silence and some mad shuffling about by all three doctors. "That's fine . . . that's what's meant to happen. No, don't . . ." Silence. "Right then, here we are . . ."

"Have you a name for the baby yet?" asked the nurse, standing next to the anesthesiologist at my head.

"Yes . . . what's going on . . . ?"

"What'll you call it, then?"

"He's John Joseph Leary, after his grandfather. . . . We're planning to call him Jack."

"Oh, I like that . . . ," the nurse began, but then she was summoned to the bottom of the table.

"Watch yourself there. . . . That's it . . . right," said Mr. Prosser.

There was silence, and then, amazingly, there was a cry. Mr. Prosser had warned me not to expect the baby to cry, as his lungs would be too weak. But he did cry out, and instantly he was no longer "the baby." He was Jack. Mr. Prosser held him above the curtain for a microsecond, and then he was whisked away to the SCBU.

I found out only later that it's pharmaceutical heroin that British doctors inject into your IV once your baby is delivered via cesarean—which would help explain the euphoria that followed. I found myself in a small room, filled with warm sunshine, which seemed odd to me, since there were no windows. Dr. Ubin entered the room and told me he had heard about the delivery.

"I know," I gushed. "I'm a mother"

"I'm sorry. I really thought he would hang in there for you."

I replied, "I've never been happier in my life." And it was true.

Dr. Ubin left, and nurses came and went. It's all a bit of a blur, but I can easily say that that recovery room stands out in my mind as one of the few places I've been where I've felt at absolute peace with the world. *I'm a mother,* I thought. *I have a son.*

AT SOME POINT I was moved to the postnatal ward, and within a few hours, in response to my constant harassment, a nurse agreed to wheel me down to the SCBU. The trip to the neonatal unit from the maternity ward takes about three minutes altogether, including the elevator ride, but I was still stoned out of my gourd, and it seemed as if it took days. I dozed off in my wheelchair as we awaited the elevator, and I had an intricately plotted dream that featured dazzling colors, music, and a cast of thousands. I awoke with the sense that I had slept for hours, but in fact I was only being wheeled into the elevator. I dozed off again and had an entire series of dreams. Warm, beautiful dreams that carried on into infinity, and when I awoke again, I was being wheeled out of the elevator into the SCBU. Now I focused on keeping my head erect and remaining awake. I was about to meet my son, but one of my eyes wouldn't stay open. It watered and slammed shut spasmodically, over and over again. I was wheeled down the corridor, through two sets of doors, and into Room A.

Even when you're drugged, the sounds of a neonatal unit are disconcerting. From the moment we entered Room A, I was enveloped in a constant symphony of beeps and alarms. I blinked at the dizzying array of machinery. Then my wheelchair spun around, and I was facing Jack, my beautiful baby boy, whom I recognized instantly. His hair (he had hair!) was flaxen blond, and I could see the swirl in the back that would later become a pesky cowlick. His nostrils flared slightly like mine, and his lips were pursed like a Kewpie doll's. His legs were long like his father's, and his chin had a handsome dimple, like Kirk Douglas's.

"Good afternoon, Mrs. Leary. My name is Ruth. I'm Jack's nurse today," said a quiet voice with a lilting West Indian accent. I turned and saw Ruth standing next to my chair, a middle-aged woman with brown skin and startlingly exquisite gray-blue eyes.

"Hi," I said. "Is he . . . okay?"

"He is doing very well. The doctor will talk to you later today, but I can say that we are all pleased he is breathing on his own. That's just a little oxygen we have blowing on him," she said, pointing to a tiny oxygen mask lying next to Jack's face.

Jack was asleep, but every few moments his forehead would furrow and his mouth would work its way into a frown, and when it did, he looked like an old man trying to recall something precious from his past. A web of wires was strung across Jack's tiny body, and Ruth patiently explained each one.

"This is the pulse oximeter," she said, pointing to a tiny light bandaged to Jack's foot. "It measures the oxygen saturation in Jack's blood. These leads go to the cardiorespiratory monitor," she said, pointing to red stickers holding wires to Jack's chest and abdomen.

"These count his heartbeats per minute and also the number of breaths he takes. You can look here," she said, pointing to a monitor, "to see what they are."

On the monitor, numbers flashed frantically, but Ruth assured me they were in the normal range. "When they go outside what is normal, an alarm sounds," she said, and no sooner were the words out of Ruth's mouth than an alarm sounded on the monitor of a tiny preemie in the isolette next to Jack's.

"Oh, my God!" I cried, waiting for Ruth to begin CPR, and I was shocked to see that she casually glanced at the baby, then flicked a switch on its monitor to stop the alarm.

"These alarms sound all the time. Usually it's simply because the baby has moved slightly." Then she said, "Would you like to have a cuddle?"

I was sure I had misunderstood Ruth, and I gave her a blank stare. Did the nurses' duties actually include cuddling distraught mothers? "We don't like to disturb the babies unnecessarily," she said, "but Jack is due for a nappy change, so you can cuddle him for a few minutes."

I told Ruth that I was on painkillers and was afraid I would drop him.

"I'll help you," she said, carefully removing his tiny diaper and replacing it with a clean one. "It's important that you hold him now. It's good for both of you."

Then Ruth lifted Jack from the table. His entire body fit into one of her hands, and with the other she gently pressed the monitor lines across his skin.

"Unbutton the top of your gown," Ruth said quietly, and I did. Then Ruth carefully placed Jack against my bare chest, and my hands instinctively went around his warm, delicate body for the very first time. I felt his vital heat against my cold, heart-pounding chest, and I remember thinking, over and over, *I'm sorry, Jack . . . I'm sorry, Jack. . . .*

"I think . . . I should put him back," I said, tears rolling down my cheeks. "I think it's too cold for him out here."

Ruth took a blanket from Jack's isolette and covered us. "Your body is keeping him nice and warm."

Then, as if she'd been reading my mind, she said, "It's not doing him harm, your cuddling him. Skin-to-skin contact with his mum is important to his development. Look at his monitor now. See how his heartbeat is stabilizing? Your breathing is reminding him to breathe."

Jack's head lay against my breast. I touched his cheek. Then I smelled his hair.

"He hears your heart," Ruth said. "He remembers that sound, and it's comforting to him now."

I kissed his head and the soft cup of his neck. My fingers moved down his legs and along the smooth soles of his tiny feet, I listened to Ruth explain about early babies in her warm Caribbean voice, and Jack listened to my heart, and gradually the sounds of the unit—the beeping and thumping and ringing—began to fade, and soon I no longer heard them at all.

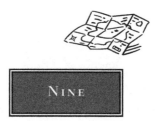

NINE

I HAD FRIENDS who had given birth by cesarean section in the United States, and I was under the distinct impression that they recovered primarily in bed, for at least a day or two. The nurses at UCH would have none of that. According to them, lying in bed after surgery was an open invitation to blood clots, infection, and bowel disorders, and the moment I lay back against my pillow those first couple of days, a cheerful powerhouse in a blue uniform would be at my side, jollying me up out of bed again.

I never felt I could whine, or say no, or complain to British nurses, and I think that had something to do with the fact that they were called "sisters," and that gave them a divine edge, in my Catholic mind. I later learned that the use of the term "sister" did have a religious origin, but the sisterhoods that became involved in nursing in Britain in the nineteenth century were Anglican, not Roman. Denis's actual sister is a nurse, and so are most of his female cousins. Until Jack was born, I thought the only thing that separated these women from me was a degree in nursing. They seemed like normal people at all the weddings and barbecues we attended, sipping their wine coolers and wiping their kids' noses. Now I know that I have as much in common with them as I do with an international spy or a death-defying stuntman. Nurses have nerves of steel and the mind-over-matter proficiency of a Buddhist monk. If, for example, you haltingly inform a nurse that you have just passed what appeared to be a large part of your brain into the toilet, via the birth canal, the nurse will not gag but instead will admonish you for flushing it away before showing it to her. Blood, phlegm, and mucus—all things intrauterine or subdermal, septic or dyspeptic—are attended to with efficient grace by nurses, who are the underpaid soothers and healers in every hospital, all over the world.

The nurses at University College Hospital wore uniforms that consisted of a navy dress topped with a crisp white apron. The dress was belted at the waist, and a name tag was pinned to the apron's breast pocket. One of the nurses told me that the type of dress and the color of belt indicated the rank of the nurse, be she ward matron, staff nurse, or nursing student. I have to say that these uniforms gave the nurses an air of professionalism that can't be conveyed in the baggy green scrubs that our American nurses wear. The British nurses also used more formal manners, and it was the first time since my marriage that I was routinely referred to as "Mrs. Leary."

One of the hardest things for me about having a baby in a neonatal unit was coming to terms with my feelings toward the staff. On the one hand, I was filled with gratitude and respect for these overworked professionals. They were my baby's saviors, and his life depended upon them, but this dependence made me feel . . . well, redundant. I had tried to produce a healthy baby, had failed horribly, and now the doctors and nurses had been forced to step in and sort out the whole mess. I felt like an actress who'd been replaced by somebody far more talented, but nobody had the nerve to tell me to get off the set. Actually, there was one staff member who I suspected might happily do the dirty deed of firing me as a parent, and that was Miss Eugenia Borthwick.

I met Miss Borthwick when Jack was a day old. I had decided to walk to the unit that morning, which took me a while due to the fresh cesarean scar, but when I arrived, I discovered that Denis had returned! I found him in three-day-old clothes, smiling into Jack's isolette. He had one hand inside, and Jack's impossibly tiny hand was actually wrapped around Denis's pinkie. One of the nurses brought me a chair, and Denis and I just sat there for a while, gazing at our son. Later that morning Denis went out to find some breakfast, and my mother was with me when Miss Borthwick appeared next to Jack's isolette. My mother was wearing her little suit and her heels, and Miss Borthwick's immediate disapproval of us was almost palpable. Miss Borthwick wore the highly starched uniform of a senior nurse. Her white-gray hair was pulled back into a tidy knot, and she carried a clipboard and a three-ring binder.

"Mrs. Leary? I'm Miss Borthwick."

"Oh. Hello," I said.

"It appears that you forgot to sign in to the unit when you came into the SCBU today."

"Um," I said. "We're supposed to sign in?"

"Yes," said Miss Borthwick, after a weighty silence.

"Oh, sorry, nobody told us."

"No, I'm sure nobody had the time. You'll notice we're quite busy most of the time, as we're seriously understaffed. Perhaps in American hospitals, nurses have time to explain ward policies to parents in person. Our nurses have all they can do administering to the needs of the babies. There's a large sign on the wall by the entrance that explains the signing-in policy."

"Oh, okay," I said, suddenly feeling as if I'd barged into Miss Borthwick's own bedroom uninvited. "I'll go sign in now."

I turned and started to limp back to the entrance, but Miss Borthwick said, "Mrs. Leary, I've brought the sign-in sheet to you. It's right here."

I thanked Miss Borthwick profusely as she handed me the clipboard. Under NAME I wrote "Ann Leary," under PATIENT I wrote "Jack Leary," and under RELATIONSHIP I wrote, with trembling fingers, "Mother."

* * *

I HAVE NEVER felt so much in the way as I did those first days in the Special Care Baby Unit. Fortunately, several of the nurses were sensitive to this. One who was particularly kind was Joan Dyer. It was Joan who told me that when a mother gives birth to a premature infant, her milk contains special nutrients not found in the milk of a mother with a full-term infant. These are nutrients that preemies are lacking and very much need. "Isn't the human body remarkable?" Joan said cheerfully, in her Belfast brogue. I can't begin to describe how empowering it was to learn that there was something I could do—that *only* I could do—to help my baby. Back upstairs on the ward, Denis was with me when a midwife arrived with the breast pump, a surprisingly large, medieval piece of metal machinery with which I would develop an intimate love/hate relationship during the months to come. The midwife showed me how to attach a piece of sterile tubing to the machine. On the other end was a suction funnel, which was placed precariously over my nipple.

My breasts are small. I don't really know how else to describe them. It seemed to me that the nipple should fit tightly into the funnel, but instead the funnel haphazardly covered almost my entire breast. "Do these things come in smaller sizes?" I asked. Then the midwife turned on the machine, and it was like I'd stuck my breast into the world's most powerful vacuum-cleaner hose. "OH, MY GOD," I said, and then I was shocked into silence as I watched milk flow from my breast and into a sterile container, destined for Jack. I had finally discovered a part of my reproductive equipment that wasn't faulty, and I beamed with pride.

"Well, what do you think about that?" I asked Denis.

"I think we'll have to take you outside for a nice graze after we're through in here, Bossy," Denis replied.

JACK WAS BORN at almost twenty-eight weeks' gestation, weighing two pounds, six ounces. The fact that he hadn't needed to be ventilated immediately after he was born was a very good thing, we were told by the neonatology staff. Jack's main problem was that his body was not mature enough for the real world. He had no suck reflex, so he received my breast milk through a tube that ran through his nose and down into his stomach. Although he could breathe on his own, his respiratory system had not developed to the point where it could regulate itself, and he routinely experienced apnea (a terrifying pause in breathing) and bradycardia (a horrifying slowing of the heart-beat). We were told that if all went well and Jack didn't develop any setbacks, such as an infection, he would be ready to leave the hospital around his due date, which was still twelve weeks away.

We had no money, but we had a plan. Denis would exchange my first-class return ticket for an economy round-trip ticket and fly back to New York. His manager had booked some comedy gigs for him, and he would stay in the States for a few weeks and work. The only hitch in the plan was that *I* needed a place to stay, and we couldn't afford even the cheapest hotel rooms in London for three months. Two days before I was due to be discharged from the hospital, one of the midwives, Beth, told us that there was a social worker in the hospital who might be able to find us emergency housing. She said that she'd spoken to the social worker about us already and had arranged to have her meet with us the next day. Beth told us that the social worker needed her to get some information from us, and that she would stop back later that day.

"What kind of information?" I asked.

"Oh, nothing really," said Beth. "She just wants to know that a real need exists."

Denis and I couldn't have felt needier.

Later, when Beth came in, Denis was gone, but my mother was with me in my room. Beth had a notebook with her, and I introduced her to my mother.

"Is this your first trip to London?" Beth asked my mother.

"Oh, no," my mother replied. "We come every year."

That's enough, Mom, I thought.

"Every year?" said Beth. "Do you have relatives here?"

Just say no, I thought. *Then don't say anything else.*

"No," my mother said. "No, we have good friends who live in Henley-on-Thames whom we visit each year. We come each June for the regatta and—"

No, this can't be happening, I thought. *She's not going to utter the words "Royal As—"*

"—Royal Ascot!"

Not exactly the picture of neediness that I had hoped to portray.

After Beth left, my mother and I took the elevator down to the SCBU.

"Mom," I said, "maybe it would be better if I meet with this social worker alone tomorrow."

"Why?"

"Because when you talk about your wealthy friends and Ascot and everything, it's likely to make her think we're rich and I can afford to stay in a hotel for three months."

"Why would she think that? What does my visiting the Thwaites with Steve have to do with you?" My mother was tired. The words came out short and hard.

"Well, you're my mother," I said shakily. "That nurse who just interviewed us probably thinks that you're married to my father and that we all go jet-setting around the world like the Kennedys, so . . ."

"Maybe it would be better if I wasn't here at all," my mother said, and we rode the rest of the way down to the unit in silence.

* * *

THE NEXT DAY I met with the social worker alone, and she told me that there are two nurses' dormitories, where some of the nursing students and residents live. One was a few blocks away, on Gower Street. The other was right across the street from the hospital on Huntley Street. There was a vacancy in the Gower Street residence now, and I could move there when I was discharged. In a week there would be a vacancy at the Huntley Street residence, and I could move and spend the rest of Jack's hospitalization there. The price was only ten pounds a night, and the only proviso was that Denis couldn't stay with me, as it was a single room. This was fine, I told her, since Denis was leaving the next day.

MY MOTHER HAD planned to stay for a week, and now she was scheduled to return home. My parents had pooled their frequent-flier miles and purchased a ticket for my sister, Meg, to come to London for a few days after my mother left. Then, after Meg left, the plan was for my father to come see me. This was a great plan in theory, but somehow, the day I was discharged from the hospital, none of my family was in London. Denis and my mother had left, and Meg wasn't due to arrive for another two days. My belongings were packed in a large blue hospital bag that had SANITATION printed in large block letters on the front, and I walked out of the Women's Hospital with the bag thrown over my shoulder like a hobo's sack. I had only two maternity outfits to wear for the next several months, and I made my way down Huntley Street swathed in an outsize tunic and leggings that I felt perfectly accented the utter deflation of body and soul I was experiencing.

I couldn't stop crying. I cried on my way to my new lodgings. Cried when the puzzled manager gave me my key, and then, when I was alone in my dorm room, I really cried. Later I was able to stop crying long enough to go see Jack, and I ran into Joan Dyer, who told me she'd found a spare breast pump I could borrow, so that I could use it at night. I was so grateful I burst into tears again. "I'll drop it off on my way home," said Joan. "It's too heavy for you with that fresh cesarean scar." Later that night Joan hauled the heavy breast pump all the way to my room on the back of her bicycle.

I started to meet some of the parents of the other, very ill babies in the unit, and I learned that preemies are usually healthiest when they are first born and that it's the stress of leaving waterworld that causes common problems such as intraventricular hemorrhages (brain bleeds), respiratory distress syndrome (collapsed lungs), and necrotizing enterocolitis (rotted intestines). Those first few days, when my mother and Denis were with me, Jack was relatively healthy, but as soon as I was discharged from the hospital, he had what the doctors called a setback. The apneas and bradycardias increased, he developed a temperature, and they began culturing his blood to determine what was wrong. Jack's little hand and foot were pricked for blood twice a day from the day he was born in order to detect infection before it was too late. Because there was so little blood in his tiny body, these blood tests made him anemic, and he needed to receive numerous blood transfusions. There were parts of his arm where the skin had been completely pulled off from the IV bandages. His blood saturation dropped, he was placed in an oxygen hood, and I was warned that he *might* need a respirator, he definitely *did* need a spinal tap, and just when I started having romantic thoughts about hurling my body into the Thames, I walked into the unit and found my dear sister, Meg, standing next to Jack's isolette.

Poor Meg. As if the shock of first seeing her tiny anemic nephew weren't enough, she now had to reckon with me, a pot-bellied, wild-eyed shell of my former self. But this is the great thing about Meg. She's an organizer. My mother and I actually think it goes beyond that and borders on obsessive-compulsive territory (you should see her cabinets), but organizing was exactly what I needed. Within hours of her arrival, Meg had assessed my requirements and had acquired bus maps, tube maps, and street maps. Maps in hand, we got on a bus and found a market and a pharmacy. Then, because my mother and Steve had generously offered to loan us money, we opened a checking account in a local bank so that they could wire it from home. Then Meg, who was only twenty-four years old and earning little more than minimum wage, took me to the Gap and bought me some jeans and T-shirts. Back at the nurses' dormitory, Meg looked at the other residents walking in and out and said, "There's a cafeteria here someplace." Upon further investigation she found the cafeteria for hospital workers and students, which was cheap enough for me to eat in every day. When we returned to the SCBU, Meg spoke with the doctors about Jack and was able to listen and actually retain information that had eluded me earlier. Later that week she helped me move from the Gower Street residence to Huntley Street, and right around then—perhaps somehow aware that Meg was a force to be reckoned with—Jack improved. His temperature dropped, and by the time Meg left at the end of the week, he was out of the oxygen hood.

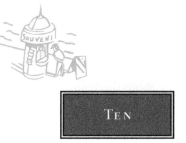

Ten

O N   T H E   E V E N I N G of my second day in the Huntley
Street residence, I decided to walk through the underground tunnel to the hospital. The social worker who'd found
my room had told me I should walk through the tunnel at night,
rather than cross Huntley Street alone. Until then, Huntley
Street had seemed perfectly benign to me, with its bright streetlights and quaint Victorian buildings, but I thought maybe there
was something I didn't know. Maybe a criminal frequented the
area, a ripper or a strangler, so I took her advice and walked
through the shabby lobby to the tunnel stairs.

There turned out to be a lot of stairs, far more, it seemed to
me, than were needed to reach an underground tunnel. When I
finally got to the bottom, I found myself at an intersection in
what I came to discover was a labyrinthine series of dimly lit

halls. I was faced with the choice of going left, right, or straight, and because I had just descended a twisting staircase, I had no idea in which direction the hospital might be. I listened for sounds from the hospital, but I heard only the hissing of water pipes. Far down the hall to the left, I could see signs posted high on the wall, so I started in that direction. Every few seconds I heard a loud clunking noise, and I held my breath and quickened my pace. My footsteps echoed above and behind me, and I tried to keep all thoughts of rats and rapists from my mind. Instead I thought about the many people who must have found shelter here in this long subterranean hall during German air raids. *This is a shelter,* I told myself, *not a tomb,* and when I arrived at the signs, I was relieved to discover that one said WOMEN'S HOSPITAL and the other said CHAPEL, both with arrows pointing in the direction I was going.

I turned a corner and saw the door marked CHAPEL. I'd been wanting to find a church since Jack was born and had been meaning to locate one close to the hospital. I imagined entering a historic cathedral and sinking to my knees in prayer. There, in the rich warmth of an aged pew, I would beseech God to spare my baby, and I was sure that I would gain some kind of understanding and perhaps be fortified by the experience.

I opened the door to the chapel. It was a small, empty room with several rows of pale wooden benches facing a stark altar. A large metal cross hung above the altar, and I gazed at it, wondering how many others had stared at this same cross with bleak questions aimed at its center. It seemed to me that this chapel was designed for mourning, this austere room in the bowels of the hospital, and that no solace could be found here for people like me, who just wanted to place requests.

I left the chapel and finally found the steps leading up to the hospital. I walked into the neonatal unit, and the crisp, antiseptic scent of rubbing alcohol, the ticking of monitors, and the smart rhythm of nurses' feet—all of it was suddenly familiar and comforting. Jack lay asleep in his isolette, his arms and legs limp and straight but his chest rising and falling. I watched him breathe as I had so many times, and after each breath I willed him to take another. *Again,* I thought over and over, and his chest rose and fell obligingly.

Whenever I arrived in the unit, I would check the clipboard that hung from Jack's isolette. It held a chart where the nurses recorded every bradycardia and apnea episode Jack experienced each hour. He got an X each time he forgot to breathe or his heart forgot to beat. Some days these things happened to Jack several times an hour, and his chart would be dark with this information. The nurses also wrote Jack's weight on the chart each day. In the beginning he lost some of his precious ounces and went down to about two pounds. Then he began to gain, and each ounce gained was like an affirmation of life itself. (*Breathe, digest, grow.* I actually tried to will Jack to do these things by staring into his glass case and thinking the words, like a chant, each time his weight went down or his heart balked too often.) If the attending nurse wasn't busy with another baby, she would give me an update on Jack's progress. One nurse who had a remarkably cheerful demeanor would say, "I'm afraid Jack was a bit naughty last night," meaning he'd had too many "bradys," and the first time she said this, I envisioned him leaping from his isolette, snatching the pen from her hand, and running down the hall shrieking with laughter, leads and monitor lines trailing behind him. I was often surprised by the way the staff talked about the babies. Doctors were always saying things like, "I've never liked this baby's lungs" or "Little Sam looks knackered. Let's up his oxygen."

Because the physical space was cramped, the parents of the babies in the unit were forced to become acquainted. Jack slept twenty-three and a half hours a day, but he was the only person I knew in England, so I basically spent my entire day at his side, gazing into his isolette. I would like to report that I immediately became the darling of the SCBU, adored by staff and parents alike, but in retrospect I think it was, for some, like having a college roommate with a serious personality disorder who never left the dorm.

Other parents had jobs, homes, and children and could sometimes spend only an hour or two with their babies. They would arrive in the unit, and there I'd be. Hints like, "You really should get out more. It would do you a world of good," and even "You still here?" were lost on me, as every time I strayed even a few blocks from the hospital, I would imagine the unit bursting into flames or Jack's heart not beating or his intestines exploding, and I would literally run back to the hospital.

Very early on, I noticed that some of the other parents in the unit were able to listen carefully to the attending nurses and physicians and had faith that these highly trained professionals knew exactly what they were doing. I, on the other hand, skimmed through every book I could find on prematurity, processed just enough information to make myself thoroughly demented with fear, and then, with my dangerously minute amount of knowledge, began to doubt and second-guess all the doctors, nurses, and carefully laid-out procedures in the unit. I worried that the medical staff was (1) overtired, (2) underpaid, and (3) not as up-to-date on current neonatal practices as I, who had just read a book called *Born Too Soon*. I also believed that the staff was filtering information in an effort to not cause alarm, so I became hypervigilant during the most mundane conversations with them.

One morning, as I was about to enter the unit, I was stopped by one of the neonatal nurses.

"Hello, Mrs. Leary," she said cheerfully. "Would you please wait outside the unit for about ten minutes while the doctors are doing their rounds."

I stood frozen in place. Through the glass wall, I saw that Jack's isolette was completely surrounded by doctors.

"You can wait in the parents' lounge if you'd like," said the nurse. Her studied calm and her casual remark about doctors' rounds were not having their intended effect, and I frantically tried to decode what I viewed as a cryptic stock phrase handed to all parents whose babies had taken a turn for the worse.

"Um . . . can I . . . ?" I couldn't finish the sentence, as I was about to burst into hysterical crying. So I stood with lips twisted into what I hoped was a smile but knew was more of a hideous grimace.

"Or . . . you could wait right here," said the nurse. Then she stepped backward slowly, as if she were afraid to turn her back on me, and I stood outside the unit peering in through the glass, anxiously studying the doctors' expressions. As it turned out, there was nothing the matter that day. The doctors make rounds each morning, and there's simply not enough room for parents to be in the unit at the same time.

It was always heartbreaking seeing a new set of parents arrive in the neonatal unit. Usually the father of the baby would get there first, while the mother recovered from the trauma of birth. Almost without fail, the father would be immediately captivated by the machinery. The valves, gauges, and beeping monitors would beckon him from the moment he set foot in the unit, and he would ask the staff a multitude of questions about the engineering and operation of these devices. *Ah,* he would think, *now everything's under control.* After the chaotic mess of the female version, which he had just so dramatically witnessed, these man-made wombs were comfortingly sterile and efficient, and by the time his wife arrived at the baby's side, he would have learned all there was to know about each device.

"Right, so here we have the pulse oximeter, or 'pulse ox,'" he would begin enthusiastically, and then he would give his wife a detailed rundown on the machine's operations, the history of its applications in neonatology, and its revolutionary effectiveness in monitoring blood-oxygen levels. The wife would blink back tears and tilt her head and try to envision her baby without tubes in its nose and wires covering its skin. She would, like me, imagine the baby in her own embrace, removed from the machine's cold, authoritative control.

Whenever a new baby appeared in the unit, I wanted to know what was wrong, and with most babies it was obvious. Either they were very premature or they had sadly visible birth defects. Every now and then, however, a healthy-looking full-term baby would show up in the unit, and I would ask the nurses why it was there. The answer was always the same: "None of your business." I have to admit that this irritated me. Because I spent so much time in the unit, I considered the nurses my friends. We discussed their boyfriends and their money problems, and some even griped about the annoying Miss Borthwick, which always thrilled me, so I felt that their sudden refusal to share information regarding these babies was a mean show of rank and power. They were nurses, and I was not.

Still, the tight confines of the space ensured that all parents eventually learned more than they wanted to know about the babies and one another. Jack's room, which held the sickest babies, was shaped like an L, and there were four other babies in his half when we arrived. First there was tiny Daniel, who was the smallest baby in the unit. He weighed just a little over a pound and was very ill. His mother and father were teenagers and seemed somehow sheltered by their ignorance. They appeared to be not altogether sure how they had gotten from a post-rave one-night stand to the Special Care Baby Unit. They smiled uncomprehendingly at doctors who told them there might be a difficult decision to be made if their baby didn't improve. If a nurse asked them to leave the unit while a procedure was being performed on their baby, these premature parents left without asking what the procedure would be.

Then there was Chloe, a six-month-old who'd been born full term with a genetic disorder that had caused a cleft palate, a cleft lip, a deformed leg, and some serious heart problems. Chloe was adored by everyone, staff and parents alike. She was developmentally normal and was the only baby in the unit who was mature enough to smile—and she was a smiler. Her mouth was terribly disfigured from the cleft palate, but she smiled beautifully with her eyes, and it was like an addictive substance that none of us could get enough of. Everyone who passed her crib spoke with her and cooed to her, and the nurses showered her with affection. Her parents, Kevin and Sara, had two other children at home, which was an hour away, and they were having financial hardships, but they came to see Chloe every day, often spending hours with her. They were veterans of the ward, and despite Chloe's frequent setbacks, they were optimists. They had complete faith in the staff, knew all the other parents, and seemed to keep in touch with graduates of the unit as well.

Another resident of the ward was Charles, who had been born at twenty-five weeks' gestation, five months earlier. Charles had been on a respirator since birth. He had respiratory distress syndrome, bronchopulmonary dysplasia, and numerous other complications that were related either to his prematurity or to the treatments he had undergone that were necessitated by the prematurity. Charles's head was swollen due to hydrocephalus, and his whole body was grotesquely enlarged from the steroids that helped him breathe. His skin seemed too tight for him, and he was on so much morphine that he was never really awake. His life had been spent in limbo. Although Charles's condition never seemed to improve, his mother, Lisa, came to see him every day. Lisa was different from most of us who had newer arrivals on the ward. She wasn't as panic-stricken, but she wasn't really normal. She had a flat affect, which might just have been her personality but was more likely the result of depression and hopelessness regarding her baby's condition.

Occasionally healthier full-term newborns were admitted to the unit for a few days for observation after a difficult birth. I had become so accustomed to the appearance of tiny preemies that these chubby babies looked like freakish giants among their delicate, lilliputian neighbors. I often found myself clucking sympathetically at the sight of these babies, until I remembered that that's how babies are supposed to look. One of them, Stephen, was a large blond baby who had inhaled some fluid during the delivery and needed oxygen. His Scottish parents had other children at home, so the mother, Jane, would come visit in the morning and the father, Angus, came on his way home from work in the evenings.

Angus was a malcontent. He would stroke his child and

glance at his chart, but most of his time in the SCBU was devoted to identifying National Health Service mismanagement and waste. Angus bitterly resented authority and treated the doctors with disdain.

"I'm sure ye've never seen a neonatal unit as pathetic as this in the United States," he said to me one day.

"I've never seen a neonatal unit at home," I replied.

"I have," said Angus. "On one of yer programs. Yer *Sixty Minutes*. American hospitals are spotless clean. Ye could eat off the floor." Then he motioned toward the floor under his baby's isolette and shook his head in disgust.

"I don't know," I said, in a voice that I hoped was loud enough for Miss Borthwick, who was just walking past, "I think the most important thing is the quality of the nursing staff. I don't think you'd find as well trained and motivated a staff in an inner-city American hospital."

Angus laughed aloud and replied, also loud enough for Miss Borthwick, "This lot motivated? You must be joking!"

Although Angus was quick to blame the staff at the SCBU for lackadaisical sanitary conditions, in my mind Jack's very existence was jeopardized by Angus's own young boys, who were brought into the SCBU each day to visit Stephen. One of the boys had a perpetually runny nose, and both children looked like they hadn't washed their hands since their mother's first trimester. I was appalled the first time they came skipping into the unit and was certain the nurse on duty would chase them out immediately. Instead she made a big fuss over them and helped each of them hold their baby brother. When they weren't peering into Stephen's isolette, they were peering into Jack's, and I started positioning myself protectively between Jack and Stephen every time the boys appeared.

"Okay, please . . . don't come too close. I wouldn't want you to catch any of Jack's germs and give them to Stephen," I would say to the boys in a trembling voice. The boys would completely ignore me and wander, deliberately breathing, all over the SCBU. One day, after the boys had gone home with their parents, I decided to approach Joan Dyer. I had thought long and hard about the most diplomatic way to present this problem.

"Joan," I began with a smile, "my sister-in-law has sent me several books about the treatment of premature babies—*American* books, you know—and, interestingly, in America they don't allow siblings of neonates into the units."

"Ah, I've heard. Shameful, really."

"Well, I can see the point, actually. See, the older children go to school and day care and could pick up all sorts of germs. Then, if they pass them on to one of the babies here, I mean their little immune systems aren't equipped yet. Where a normal newborn might be able to fight off viruses, these little ones . . ."

Joan was a senior nurse. She had gone through four years of college, followed by four years of nursing school and then two more years of specialized schooling in neonatology. She had nursed hundreds of babies in this SCBU over the years, and now she was being issued a lesson on the immunology of neonates by me, the learned reader of a *single* book about preemies. Joan stood patiently and listened as I explained about the masks and gowns that Americans are required to wear in neonatal units. She nodded as I described the mandatory scrubbing of hands that parents are required to do before they may touch their babies.

When I'd finished, Joan said, "Is that right? Do they still make parents wear masks to visit their own babies in the States?"

"Yes," I replied, relieved. I was getting through.

"Interesting. You know, that's considered very old-fashioned here. We stopped doing that years ago. There was a study done, and it was discovered that babies in neonatal units don't usually become infected by germs from their family members. It's mostly the doctors and nurses, carrying germs from one baby to another, who cause problems. The study also revealed that the masks and gowns and gloves cause a serious psychological barrier between the infant and the parents, and sometimes this can cause problems with bonding."

Joan then cited studies proving that babies who are overly protected from germs in SCBUs don't develop the necessary resistance to infections and are more ill in subsequent years than babies who've been in neonatal units with more relaxed standards. Joan's explanations made sense, and I was certain she would end the conversation by saying, "In the future do you mind keeping your big trap shut about things pertaining to the operation of this unit? We have things very well in hand, as you can see." Instead Joan placed her hand on my arm. "I don't know how you parents cope with all the worry. I really don't. Keep pumping your breast milk for Jack. That's the best protection he can have."

VERY EARLY ONE morning, when Jack was just a couple of weeks old, I arrived in the unit to find that Stephen had gone home and a new baby, Alexander, had moved in next to Jack. Seated beside his isolette was a pretty young woman with long auburn hair. She was reed thin and wore trendy low-slung jeans and a tight-fitting top. We said hello and introduced ourselves—her name was Faith—and when I admired her handsome, full-term baby, she informed me that she had just delivered him earlier that morning. I was taken aback by this information. This woman's baby weighed over eight pounds, but to look at her, you would never have known she'd been pregnant. Jack, on the other hand, weighed two and a half pounds, but looking at my body, you might suspect that he had a morbidly obese twin awaiting a later delivery date.

Faith's intense beauty and mysterious ways were a source of constant fascination for me. She was as lean as a greyhound, but she swilled Coke and ate chocolate biscuits at six-thirty in the morning. Her handsome husband, who arrived later with their toddler, shared her casual demeanor and her affinity for candy and soft drinks. Faith spoke to her little boy, Max, in a calm, soothing manner. Max had a gorgeous round, pale face surrounded by light brown curls, and he would say things like, "May I have a biccy, Mummy?" or "May I give Alexander a cuddle now?" This child didn't whine but spoke in such a sweet, plaintive voice that sometimes I'd blurt out, "Of course you can!" before his mother had a chance to answer.

Faith and I became friends, and we spent many hours admiring our babies and expressing milk together. I liked Faith, despite the fact that in her delicate presence I felt like a large, lumbering hillbilly. Faith's movements were graceful and cat-like. Walking beside her one day, I remembered that when I was a child, kids used to tease me about my walk, which is more of a saunter, really, as my shoulders and head are overly involved in each stride. Faith met each day with a serene, almost other-worldly calm, which I attributed to the Buddhism she told me that she and her husband practiced. Panicked mania was my overriding emotional condition, and I wanted what Faith had. Sometimes, while seated in the parents' lounge, Faith would seem to be in a meditative state, and I would close my eyes as well and try to visualize myself walking along a warm, tropical beach. Unfortunately, I could manage only a couple of steps before my psyche would be catapulted back to cold, scary London, where my very ill baby was hospitalized.

One thing that worried me about Faith was that she seemed unclear about what exactly was wrong with her baby. She would say things like, "I thought they were going to let me bring him home today, but now they want to observe him for another two days." I would ask why, and she would shake her head and shrug. I was certain that the baby was fatally ill with a heart condition and the doctors were not being straightforward with Faith. Because she was quite young, I decided to take her under my wing. "You have to ask questions," I would gently encourage her. "You're his advocate. Ask the doctors why they're holding your baby," I would say over and over, and she would bite her lip and nod. After the doctors finished their rounds each day, I'd tell Faith, "Don't let them leave. Go ask them why Alexander can't go home today. Go on! Ask them why!"

Finally, when Faith left the unit one day, Kate, one of the Irish nurses, said, "Jee-sus, when will you stop harassing the poor girl about her baby?"

"I'm just trying to help her," I explained.

"Help her do what?" asked Kate.

"Well," I replied, "she doesn't seem to understand what's wrong with her baby. I think sometimes the English aren't aggressive enough when it comes to demanding their rights as patients, or as parents of patients."

Then, seeing that I had Kate's rapt attention, I added, "Faith is such a natural mother that this whole hospital environment is extremely disturbing to her, and she's sort of had to zone herself out in order to deal with the stress of it all. I understand Faith," I said, "and I just want to help her get some straight information from the staff here on exactly what is wrong with her child."

"That's very interesting," replied Kate. "However, if you really understood yer friend Faith, you'd be aware that she knows perfectly well what's wrong with her baby. He was born addicted to heroin, and he's being weaned off it through the methadone in his mum's breast milk."

Unfortunately, this experience is a sad but accurate example of my pitiable abilities at character assessment. I am constantly mistaking shyness for arrogance, for example, and in this instance I mistook a junkie for a highly evolved spiritual guide.

I DID GLEAN an interesting fact about the SCBU from Kate that day. She informed me that a large three-ring binder that sat on the nurses' stand, in plain view, was used by the nurses to jot down their observations of the parents, and their inter-actions with their babies. In a case like Faith's, a social worker would review the documents before making a deci-sion about whether the baby should be allowed to go home with the mother. Faith was being scrutinized closely, Kate confided. She would have been allowed to take the baby home already, if it weren't for the fact that she'd been spotted "pinching" syringes from the doctor's cart the day after the baby's birth. I was less interested in Kate's crime report than I was in the fact that the notebook contained observations about me and my suitability as a parent. I suddenly realized that most of my time in the unit had been spent either crying or sharing my paranoid thoughts with the medical staff. I imagined an entry:

Leary mother arrived quite early and, as usual, insisted on peering in through the window during doctors' rounds. Depression and lack of sleep evident. Again displays unhealthy preoccupation with babies who are not her own. DO NOT leave her unattended in unit. Discusses feelings of guilt and inadequacy with attending nurse. Staff has experienced difficulty persuading this mother to put her baby back in isolette after holding him. Be firm.

I recalled confiding to a young nurse that I blamed myself for Jack's prematurity, and I wondered now if she thought this meant I had spent my last days of pregnancy in a crack house. I thought about my interactions with Denis, around the time of Jack's birth:

Serious marital problems evident. Mother clearly despises father. Perhaps all men. Very likely a lesbian. DO NOT allow yourself to be alone with mother. Make sure other staff are in earshot at all times.

I soon got into the habit of casually standing next to the nurses' station when I arrived at the unit. "I don't want to be in anybody's way," I'd say to the nurse. "I'll just stand over here." Then, when she was busily inserting somebody's nasal gastric tube, my eyes would slowly turn downward toward the open notebook, and I'd frantically skim through the nurses' notes, looking for any references to me or Jack. One day Miss Borthwick surprised me by dryly asking if I could pass her the notebook when I was finished reading it. I passed it to her, red-faced, and that was the last I saw of it. I imagined that day's entry went something like . . .

> This woman's behavior is abnormal, if not pathological, even taking into consideration the cultural differences (she is an American; arrogance, perversity, ignorance are to be expected to a certain degree). DO NOT leave notebook in unit anymore.

My worrying and questioning and harassing of the staff was exhausting, and each night I would return to the nurses' home and go straight to sleep. Usually around two in the morning, I would awaken drenched in postnatal sweat, breasts painfully engorged, to hear a wild party in the next room. I would insert one of my udders into the breast pump and wonder if my baby was going to live or die, and I would express, usually, more tears than milk. I would waddle down the hall, passing young couples "snogging" drunkenly, and put the expressed milk into the communal refrigerator, next to cans of beer. Then, as I tried to go back to sleep, I would pray that there would be no sirens, but as I was next to a hospital there always would be, and suddenly the *weee-a, weee-a, weee-a* World War II–movie sirens would sound. Then my sense of alienation would be complete.

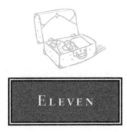

ELEVEN

WHEN I WAS a teenager, my brother, sister, and I spent every Christmas with my mother, and then a day or two later, we would take the train from Boston to Stamford, Connecticut, to visit my father. When we arrived, we would grab our bags and shuffle uncomfortably out onto the platform. We knew what was coming, and, sure enough, we immediately heard a two-fingered whistle followed by "*Halloo!*"

Our eyes would scan the parking lot until we saw him stepping slowly toward us, tripping over rubbish and walking into cars, one eye sealed to the viewfinder as if by suction, the opposite half of his face swept up into a giant squint. Although in those days my father's video camera was the size and weight of a large suitcase filled with cement, he shouldered its heft with the proud determination of Atlas himself.*

We usually stood there on the platform for a moment, frozen with stage fright. Then my father would beckon us toward him, and we'd make our way down the steps, smiling and waving into the camera. Eventually our smiles would fade and we would stop waving, but my father was always intent upon videotaping an entire sequence. If he picked us up at the train, he liked to show us walking all the way to the car, so he walked along— several feet away from us, silently indicating where the car was parked.

Always, before we reached the car, my father would clear his throat and ask, *"How was the trip?"* in the grand, stagy voice he used when he knew he could be heard on tape.

"All right, I guess," "Good," "Fine," were our mumbled replies.

"Good, good," Dad would emote. *"Everybody's waiting for you back at the house!"*

Back at the house, Terry and her three boys were, as scripted, waiting for us. Before we had a chance to open the car doors, my father would leap from the driver's seat, camcorder in hand, and videotape his wife and her children waving from the porch.

---

*My father was and is an electronics freak. I think it's possible that he was one of the first private citizens to own a video camera. It was the giant, prehistoric model available in the late seventies.

"Halloo! They're here!" he'd announce.

"Hi, come in!" Terry said, directly into the camera, and then my father turned the camera on us as we filed self-consciously into the house.

My father adored Terry's sons, and now, looking back, I can see why they might have been, at that time, slightly more appealing to my father than his biological children were. For one thing, they were younger, still in that sweet, wet-behind-the-ears stage during which teachers and parents are admired. We had graduated to that unattractive teenage stage during which all adults are viewed with derision and our worlds revolved around our friends, our clothes, and the acquisition of cigarettes and any controlled substances we could get our clammy little hands on. Also, Terry's kids had another sire, so their quirks and shortcomings were more easily overlooked by my father, who could enjoy them without any guilt or feelings of accountability. But I think what made parenting most rewarding for my father during his second marriage was the availability of the camcorder.

The video camera gave my father something he had been seeking all his years of fathering: control. When the camera was turned on, he could manipulate the behavior of everybody in his presence. We, his subjects, learned not to complain or whine, because it would be so unpleasant having to view the behavior later on. Instead we would move about in an altered, camera-ready fashion, careful not to swear or, in my case, speak at all. The sound of my recorded voice never ceases to horrify me.

(The nasality is so severe that, listening to it, one might imagine it's my nostrils moving rather than my lips.)

We hated the video camera, my brother, sister, and I, but Terry and her kids seemed not to mind it at all. The boys acted completely normal when it was turned on them, occasionally hamming it up with a sight gag like pretending they were vomiting onto each other's food, and Terry always smiled pleasantly when the camera was turned on her. When it was turned on us, we sat stone-faced, unable to think of anything to say or do that would be worth having to watch at the mandatory viewing session after lunch.

"First presents," my father would say as we sat down to a lunch of taco salad. "Then, since you couldn't spend Christmas Day with us, we videotaped it for you, so we'll watch that!"

After lunch we were herded into the family room, and as Paul and Meg and I started to flop down on the couch, my dad cried out, "No, no, kids! Over here. I've got everything set up."

In the center of the room was a tripod holding the video camera, which now was fitted out with lights. The lights beamed down on three chairs in the opposite corner of the room. "Go on!" my father said. "You kids sit over there."

We sat in the stiff dining-room chairs, side by side, and Terry laid our Christmas presents before us. Then my father turned on the camera, and we could see nothing but the bright lights boring into our eyeballs.

"Go on! You first, Meg." My father's voice could be heard from someplace behind the camera.

"Open the one with the pink wrapping, Meg! That's for you!"
Terry would chime in from what sounded like the direction of
the sofa. She, too, had a special home-video voice she sometimes used.

Meg would open her present and hold it up for the camera.
"Great sweater! Thanks . . . Dad? Terry?" Meg couldn't see
them, so she started to rise.

"No, stay there!" Dad's voice was now a stage whisper. *"You're
welcome!"* he then boomed for the benefit of the camera.

"I have something for you, it's in my backpack." Again Meg
tried to stand.

"No, we'll open ours after you kids have opened yours," my
dad whispered. *"Ann, you're next!"*

The camera made my father a director of sorts. It removed
him from the scene, from the action, and put him in the role of
creator. "Climb under the tree and get that present, Matty," my
father would whisper to his youngest stepson. "Now give it to
Paul—go on!" Matty would hand my brother the present, Paul
would give Matty a friendly pat on the shoulder, and my father
would have a moment to view later, and for eternity. It really
didn't matter to him that the moment was something he had
exploited. The unbridled randomness of family life was too
much for my father, and the viewfinder was his way out. He
taped, edited, stored, and archived his family, but later, when
we watched these tapes, along with the tapes of Terry's boys'
baseball practice, birthday parties, and their family trip to Cape
Cod, they're all present but somehow not focused completely

on what they are doing. Instead their every movement and all their words are performed for the benefit of my father, who, in all our family videos, is just a disembodied voice.

MY FATHER'S FLIGHT arrived in London at five in the morning, and he took a taxi directly to the hospital. I wasn't there yet, so one of the staff nurses led him over to Jack's isolette. Then, security being absolutely nonexistent in that SCBU, the nurse took my father at his word that he was related to Jack and asked if he would like to hold his grandson. My father asked if he shouldn't first put on a gown and mask, since he had just gotten off an international flight where the man in front of him had coughed for five solid hours, but the nurse said he should just wash his hands. Then she said, chuckling, "You Americans are so funny about germs."

When I arrived in the unit, my father greeted me warmly. Then he handed Jack to me and began examining the machinery and the monitors carefully. He watched me hold Jack for a while and listened to me recount every burp and bowel movement the baby had made since his birth, and then, I think, he saw the next four days stretching out before him—four days in an exciting foreign city, watching his daughter hold a tiny, sleeping baby—and his mission was to get us as far away from the hospital as possible, for as long as possible, every day.

"Let's go to Covent Garden," he said. "I'll buy you lunch."

I remember looking up at him from my little chair next to Jack's isolette. Lunch? Jack couldn't go to lunch. What could my father be thinking?

"Why don't you go?" I replied. "Jack usually wakes up for a few seconds this time of day. I really should be here."

One of the neonatal nurses, no doubt desperate to be relieved of my constant, depressing company, said, "Oh, for heaven's sake! That's why *we're* here. Go on, now, it'll do you good to get out with your dad for a little while. Go on!" So, after I bade Jack a teary farewell, we started down Gower Street toward Covent Garden, my father and I.

Outside, in the pale gray light of a London morning, it occurred to me that my father looked different. He seemed thinner, his forehead less furrowed, and after some time I finally realized what it was. My father didn't have his video camera with him. I had seen him frowning into a viewfinder for so many years that I'd almost forgotten what he looked like without it.

"Dad, where's your video camera?" I asked.

"Well . . . ," he began, and then he sighed and shook his head sadly. "I decided to leave it at home. I didn't have a converter. I thought still pictures would be enough, but as soon as I saw Jack, I wished I had it."

"Oh," I replied.

"I'm sorry," he said. "I didn't have any way to charge it—the voltage is different here—and those darn batteries only last about an hour."

"That's okay," I said.

"You won't think so later, when you want to see what he looked like when he was just born."

"I don't know if I'll want to see all this later. It's bad enough now," I said, but my dad wasn't listening. He had suddenly stopped walking.

"Will ya get a load of those nuts up ahead?" he said, nodding toward two college students with spiky pink hair and dog collars. "Let's cross the street."

"What? Why?" I asked, but my dad was already halfway across the street, and I was forced to follow him.

"You'll wanna keep your eyes open. This doesn't look like the best neighborhood," my father informed me.

I looked around at the beautifully kept buildings with flowers freshly planted in the window boxes. Striding past us were businessmen, construction workers, and the occasional mother pushing a stroller.

"Dad, this is a perfectly nice neighborhood . . . ," I started to explain, but when I turned to look at him, he was glaring at a pair of Islamic women walking toward us, dressed in full burqas.

"Crazy, crazy people around here," my father whispered to me as they passed.

"Those women aren't crazy, Dad. They're Muslims," I said, but what I thought was, *Who is this man?* and I realized that I had not spent more than fifteen minutes alone with my father in my entire life.

"Look, here comes a real English bobby!" my father exclaimed as a cop approached on foot. "I knew I was going to regret not bringing the camcorder. Terry would have gotten a real kick out of that!"

We waited for a bus, and when it came, my father said, "Darn it! A double-decker! Now, *that*, I would really like to have on tape." We climbed on board and rode to Covent Garden, where my father was forced to look longingly at all the American and Japanese tourists who were viewing the marketplace through the lens of a camcorder.

My father stayed in London for several days, and I was grateful for his company and also for the opportunity to observe him unfettered by the video camera. It was fascinating, for example, to listen to his frequent lamentations about what he wished he could be taping. These were always the most overly photographed and televised British scenes: a double-decker bus, the changing of the guard, the black London taxis speeding around tight corners—everything he had seen a million times, my father wanted the opportunity to record himself.

"Damn it!" he exclaimed as we watched a tourist being swarmed by pigeons in Trafalgar Square. "*That,* Terry would really get a kick out of!"

Faced with sights that really make London unique and exciting—a young man dressed in a tailored business suit staggering drunk and bloody through Central London in broad daylight, for instance—my father's eyes would dart about for something—anything—else to watch. He wanted to view things that supported his ideas of the English as a quaint, intelligent, gentle race, but he found most aspects of their lifestyle . . . well, "crazy." He repeatedly announced that the system of driving on the left-hand side of the road was "crazy." The British currency, lacking a paper pound note, was "crazy, absolutely crazy." And the prices, everywhere, were "just plain crazy."

The other interesting thing I learned about my father is that he has a remarkably high shame threshold. Take, for instance, his habit during that visit of suddenly, and loudly, speaking with what he believed was a good stab at an English accent.

"Look, there's Buckin'am Palace. Maybe we'll catch a glimpse of the queen mum 'erself, or Prince Chahls!" my father would say as we rode past in a city bus, and although in his mind he sounded like an Englishman, in fact he was doing a dead-on impersonation of the Lucky Charms leprechaun. "Ah, he's a right jolly ol' chap, that Chahls!" my father would chuckle, digging his elbow into my arm and winking at the other people on the bus, who stared at him in astonishment.

When it was time for him to return to the United States, my father made one last visit with me to see Jack in the SCBU. Jack was sleeping in his isolette, so we stood watching him silently. Again, as I had many times during that visit, I longed to see the camcorder cradled in my father's arms, not because I wanted him to videotape Jack but because without it we were all too exposed. Good-byes were always videotaped by my father, but now, within a few moments, we would bid each other farewell without the camera between us, and we both felt vulnerable and defenseless.

"Look," my father said, pointing at Jack. "His eyes are starting to blink . . . good God, they're opening! Why in God's name didn't I bring my camcorder?" he said, and then he lowered his head to get a good look at Jack's face.

Jack's eyes blinked, and then it honestly appeared that he was gazing up at my father.

"I wonder if they can see," my father said. "What can they see?"

"I think just vague shapes and shadows," I said, and now I was leaning in, staring into Jack's eyes, my face pressed close, almost touching my father's, and it really seemed then that Jack was looking right back at us.

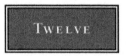

TWELVE

THE PREMATURE INFANT, in some ways, is like the prehistoric aquatic creature who has not quite evolved into a land dweller. His body is not yet equipped to deal with gravity and the wildly fluctuating temperatures of the surface world. The parts of his brain that coordinate the intricate timing of respiration have not fully developed, nor have the reflexes that enable him to suck. I suppose the hard realities of the extrauterine world come as a bit of a shock to all newborns, but full-term babies arrive equipped to survive out of water. Jack did not.

In 1902 Dr. J. W. Ballantyne, a lecturer in midwifery and gynecology at the Medical College for Women in Edinburgh, Scotland, said of the premature infant:

He is like some dweller in the hot plains of India who has been transported in a moment of time on some "magic carpet of Tangu" to the chill summits of the "frosty Caucasus"; with no opportunity for acclimatization such as a gradual transit affords, he is suddenly submitted to the severe strain which so marked a change in surroundings entails; it is possible that the marvellous adaptive mechanisms of the human body will overcome the difficulties of adjustment of capabilities to requirements, but there will be danger till this condition of physiological equilibrium is reached.

It was that ever-present sense of danger I found most harrowing about having a baby in a neonatal unit. It was like watching my child walk through a minefield and knowing exactly where the mines were hidden but not being able to tell him where they were. These hidden "mines"—infections, hemorrhages, and pulmonary disorders—had already brought down some of the other little inhabitants of the SCBU, and all I could do was sit back and hope and pray that Jack wouldn't be stricken as well.

As the days and weeks passed, Jack and I slowly began to adapt to our new worlds. Jack's body was learning to adjust to the air-breathing, gravity-bound realities of earth life, while I was unconsciously starting to incorporate words like "nappy" and "pram" into my vocabulary. I began to forget about my fantasy pregnancy, and I think Jack slowly let go of his warm memories of womb life, and we started to accept our predicament.

One factor that helped me gain this acceptance was the slow realization that we had been incredibly fortunate to have stumbled into one of the best hospitals for obstetrics and neonatology in the world. Later, when we returned to the United States, Jack's pediatricians would look at his records and ask incredulously, "Did you actually meet Dr. Reynolds?"

"Sure," I replied. Professor Reynolds, as he was called by the UCH staff, was always wandering in and out of the SCBU. He was a rather bedraggled-looking older fellow, and I assumed that he was an indulged academic eccentric from the university. In fact, Professor Reynolds is considered to be one of the most important pioneers in modern neonatology, and most neonatology students in American medical schools have studied his work.

Also, I learned that the betamethasone shots I received before Jack was born, which helped him develop surfactant in his lungs, had not yet been approved by the American Food and Drug Administration. When I returned to the United States, Jack was involved in follow-up programs with other low-birthweight preemies, and none of the other parents could believe that Jack had never been on a respirator. Had he been born in the United States, undoubtedly he would have needed ventilation and would have suffered some of the unavoidable lung complications caused by the respirator.

I was slowly adapting to the daily stresses of having a baby in an intensive-care unit, but since the very moment of Jack's birth, another change had been taking place for me. I was morphing into a besotted she-beast, a "mommy," and the intensity of this new feeling—this dizzying, heart-bursting love I felt for my baby—was something I tried to resist at first. I cried to Denis the night after Jack's birth that I was afraid to fall too much in love with Jack, because then he might die, and I didn't think I could bear it. This is the kind of thinking that baffles Denis, who is, people are often surprised to learn, an unshakable optimist. "You already love him," Denis said. "You'll love him forever anyway, whether he lives or dies. Don't try to protect *yourself*, for Christ's sake. *Jack* needs us." I knew that Denis was right, and so I surrendered to the waves of love and fear that washed over me the instant I laid eyes on our baby, every single time I saw him, and eventually the fear began to fade.

One day an elderly woman was visiting a baby in the SCBU. Her great-grandson, who had been born at full term with complications, was in an isolette near Jack.

"Oh, he's a dear little one, that," the old woman clucked when she saw me gazing at Jack in his isolette. "How much does he weigh?"

"He's about two and a half pounds," I said.

"Oh. Just like me, Mary," she said to her granddaughter, who was holding her whopping seven-pounder.

"What?" I asked.

"Granny was only a little over two pounds when she was born," said the granddaughter proudly.

"You were?" I exclaimed. "Well, that must have been . . ."

"Eighty-two years ago," said Granny.

"Wow," I said, suddenly scrutinizing the woman's appearance for defects. She looked totally normal. "Were you born in a London hospital?"

"No. We lived in the country. I was born in my mother's bed. They kept me in a box under the stove. Fed me with an eyedropper, they did!"

A smile spread across my face then, and I felt like hugging this healthy old woman. For the very first time, I thought that Jack might live, not just today or until the end of the week but for eighty years or more.

ONE AFTERNOON I arrived in the unit to find that a camera crew had crowded itself into the tight space. Miss Borthwick informed me that the crew was from ITV, a British television news station. That day members of Parliament were set to vote on whether or not legal abortion should be permitted as late as twenty-eight weeks' gestation. Because Jack had been born at twenty-eight weeks, they were wondering if they could film him for that evening's news. Denis's family was desperate to see Jack, so I consented, asking if they would give me a copy of the tape to send home.

A petite blond female reporter spoke into the camera outside the unit, and then the cameraman quickly filmed Jack lying sound asleep in his isolette. As they were packing up their equipment, I took my spot in the chair next to Jack's isolette, and the reporter approached.

"Hello," she said, smiling and extending her hand. "Are you Jack's mum?"

"Yes, hi, I'm Ann," I said.

"I'm Jo Andrews," she said warmly.

Jo thanked me for allowing them to feature Jack in their spot. Then she asked me what part of America I was from.

"Boston," I replied.

"Do you live in London now?" asked Jo.

These questions had become so familiar from other parents and visitors to the unit who recognized my accent that I entertained the idea of typing up a fact sheet and taping it on Jack's isolette.

"No," I said. "We were here on holiday, and I went into preterm labor."

Yes, I had adopted some English phrases of my own. It just seemed easier to say we were "on holiday" now, for some reason.

"Where is Jack's dad?" Jo asked.

"He's in New York. Working."

Then Jo asked a series of rapid-fire questions about the type of labor and delivery I had endured, where I was staying and how much longer Jack would be in the SCBU. When she had satisfied her journalist's mind by finding out every fact about our situation, she declared, "This is horrible!" and instantly Jo took me under her wing.

Jo had given birth to her baby daughter, Florence, six months prior, right there at UCH. She'd had a difficult delivery, and she was a new mother passionate about mothering. I think those facts contributed to her interest in helping me, but I think mainly that Jo represents all that is truly great about the English. Generosity, kindness, and loyalty had been bred into her, and once she was aware of my plight, she was constitutionally incapable of simply wishing me luck and getting on her with her life. Instead she stopped into the unit nearly every day to see how I was doing. She and her husband, Paul Walker, repeatedly invited me to their home. Jo found out about Nippers for me, a British support group for parents of premature babies. She took me out to lunch and to the House of Commons to view Question Time with Prime Minister Margaret Thatcher. Jo took me to the Chelsea Flower Show and to Camden Market. She became, instantly, a dear friend, a fierce advocate on my behalf, and my own personal tour guide.

Jo and I were both new mothers, but the similarity ended just about there. Although Jo was only a couple years older, I couldn't help feeling that she was an adult and I was not. Jo and Paul had successful careers. They owned a home. They drove a minivan that had a car seat in it for Florence. What had I been thinking? I'd often wonder after an afternoon at Jo's. Why hadn't we waited until we had a savings account before deciding to have a child? Why hadn't we done the mature, responsible thing and shown some restraint? The answer, I knew, was that I thought the day might never come when we could better afford a child. Also, in the back of my mind were two very American notions: If not now, when? And anything is possible.

I have met very few people in my life who are more suited to their occupation than is Jo, who has the inquisitiveness of a precocious child and the determination of a pit bull terrier. Jo absolutely must find out the answers to questions, and when she does, she's able to dumb down the information so that even a dull-witted American like me might understand it.

Jo brought me up to date on the current political news. When I asked her about the poll tax, which seemed to dominate the news that spring, she explained that in the late 1980s Margaret Thatcher's Tory Party had resolved itself to reform the system of collecting local taxes. They decided that the best way to do this was to introduce a poll tax, which was an identical sum to be paid by all members of a community, regardless of their income and landholdings. Residents would be taxed by their local councils rather than by the national government. What happened was that many councils considerably raised their tax rates, which meant that while wealthy landowners still paid significantly less than they had prior to the poll tax, many working- and middle-class citizens saw their tax rates skyrocket. Not surprisingly, the poll tax was wildly unpopular. Jo explained that the day of the poll-tax riots (when Denis had to make his way through bleeding mobs of angry protesters) had started out peacefully. Thousands of people had descended on Trafalgar

Square to listen to speakers denouncing the poll tax. When mounted members of the city's riot squad moved in, the crowd grew violent.

It wasn't until Jo appeared on the scene that I realized how desperately I was in need of a friend. Jo was very interested in the goings-on at the SCBU, and she filled in some of the cultural gaps for me, such as why I was starting to feel an undercurrent of resentment from some of the other parents and hospital staff.

One afternoon I was in the SCBU chatting with Chloe's mother, Sara, and Lynn, one of the nurses. Sara asked me if Jack was eligible for British citizenship, and I replied that from what I understood, he was not. Lynn confirmed this.

"It used to be that anybody born in the United Kingdom was automatically granted citizenship, but because of the huge amount of immigrants we've had in recent years, the laws have changed."

Then she said, "Still, you don't have to be a British citizen to benefit from the same services that British taxpayers are entitled to."

"Hmmm," I replied, gazing into Jack's isolette.

"After all," said Lynn, "you must think yourself very lucky to have been here in England when you went into labor with Jack. British hospitals are not allowed to turn away patients. Whether they're tax-paying citizens or not, if they walk into an NHS hospital, they will receive free treatment."

I had heard this tune before. When I was in the antenatal

unit, one of the other mothers had asked me how it felt to get free medical care for a change, leaving me to wonder how many others considered me a freeloader.

"You know," I said to Lynn, "the NHS is billing my insurance company for Jack's and my hospitalization. We're not getting free care."

"Yes," said Lynn. "But even if you had *no* insurance, you'd receive exactly the same care you're receiving now. If I was on holiday in America, and I went into labor like you did, I don't carry insurance, so I'd be out of luck, wouldn't I?"

"No," I replied. "American hospitals are also required to take emergency patients, regardless of their ability to pay. American hospitals, especially in the cities, are filled with citizens and noncitizens who have no insurance."

Lynn and Amy gave each other a look, and I realized that just as Americans tend to believe, wrongly, that socialized medicine leads to substandard health care, many Europeans believe that uninsured people in America are denied any access to doctors. They seem to envision women giving birth on the streets, children amputating their own limbs, and people blithely stepping over the sick and dying as they walk to work.

Later, having tea with Jo, I said, "I actually get the feeling that some people at the hospital think it was some kind of opportunistic scheme of mine to have Jack born here, at the expense of the British."

"Don't worry about what people say," Jo insisted. "The National Health Service is going broke, and it's a touchy subject for many, especially those who are employed by it. The whole institution has been so understaffed, underloved, and underfinanced that the inmates have gone pretty much mad. That said, I believe, as do most of my fellow Brits, that it's still the best universal health service around."

"Besides," she added, "I do think it was rather clever of you to rupture that amniotic sac at will."

PART THREE

———

The Ugly
American

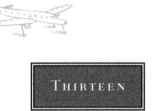

Thirteen

𝒟ESPITE MY HOMESICKNESS and uneasiness at being foreign, I felt increasingly secure in the hands of Britain's National Health Service. I began to view the NHS as a maternal entity that, while not necessarily clutching me to her bosom, was nevertheless firmly committed to the nurturing care of Jack and me. This cosy feeling of security evaporated, however, the minute I stepped outside the hospital.

For one, I never quite got over the nagging suspicion that my watchful presence was the only thing that galvanized Jack's pulmonary system. I feared that the minute my back was turned, his heart and lungs would decide that while the cat's away, the mice shall play, and they would kick back and relax a little. Sometimes I would be almost out the door and then suddenly be compelled to turn on my heel and sprint back to the SCBU.

I imagined I would find Jack's monitors blasting and the nurses trying to prod Jack's chest back into service, but of course this was usually not the case. Slowly I came to understand that Jack's body, and the SCBU as a whole, functioned just as well with or without my hovering presence.

There was something else, though. While the hospital had become my home and seemed very, very real, whenever I tried to leave I had the uneasy sense that I had penetrated the "fourth wall" and was now a character in one of my favorite films. The taxis and double-deckers and streetlights and phone booths all seemed to be carefully arranged by a set designer, and in the beginning I wouldn't have been surprised to find Dick Van Dyke leading a dancing gang of chimney sweeps down Huntley Street.

Despite my protests, the nurses began strongly encouraging me to get out and about more, and, as NHS employees, they knew what it was like to live in London on a fixed budget and were able to steer me toward free or cheap attractions. After my food and rent money, I was left with only a couple of pounds for diversions, but fortunately most of London's museums are free and their public-transit system is very inexpensive and efficient.

I had been in London several weeks before I discovered that Regents Park is only a ten-minute walk from the hospital, and almost every day I wandered through its gardens. Regents Park is beautiful. I don't know of an American park to compare with it. Central Park, which I love, has great trees and ponds and interesting rock formations, but Central Park, especially on weekends, is a bustling, energetic place. Comparatively, Regents Park is quiet and serene. The grass is impeccably maintained. You can sprawl out on it without a blanket or chair, and when you stand, there will be nothing stuck to you but a few grass clippings. No cigarette butts or condoms to brush off your clothes. Most people walk quietly in London's parks. Many, I noticed that spring, not only admired the beautifully planted flower beds but actually studied them, sometimes even jotting down notes.

I usually went to the park at the time each morning when the doctors made their rounds in the unit, and I often saw the same people each day: the elderly couple tossing bread crumbs to the rioting geese, the attractive mother with her two little boys heading for the playground, or the nurse pushing an old man around in a wheelchair. Of course there would be groups of boisterous tourists and sometimes kids cutting school, but for the most part Regents Park was an oasis of tranquillity, a place for contemplation, and, I thought, probably similar to what Frederick Law Olmsted had in mind when he designed Central Park.

Central Park, in those pre-Giuliani days, was a place where one might go to contemplate . . . the decline of the human race. As you entered the park, at least from the Seventy-second Street entrance on the West Side, you first encountered what Denis called Drunkards Row—benches lining both sides of the sidewalk—where encrusted and befungused men in various stages of undress would sleep, drink, masturbate, and still find the time to greet young women with hearty gestures and guttural propositions. A short distance ahead, you had to somehow navigate Park Drive, which, on weekends, was a mad runaway river of humanity. Bicyclists, roller skaters, joggers, unicyclists—basically anything that could move of its own volition at speeds exceeding thirty miles an hour made its way along that drive, paying no attention to traffic signals. Crossing was treacherous. (I once saw a small child who stepped off the curb and was swept up by the leg of a skater. Flailing desperately for his mother's outstretched hand, the tot was carried, plastered to the skater's leg, at least a hundred yards down the drive before his frenzied mother could rescue him.) Once you successfully crossed Park Drive, you found yourself in the very heart of things. The Great Lawn spread before you, bejeweled with litter and dog waste. Sweatshirt-hooded men sidled up to you, regardless of your age, and offered "smoke," "sense," and "X" with the tenacious goodwill of all salesmen whose supply never meets demand. Oh, the rats, the cries of gay lovers from the woods—these were the sights and sounds of Central Park in 1990, so it's no wonder that when I entered Regents Park, I often felt as if I had jumped into one of Bert's sidewalk paintings in *Mary Poppins*.

In London people walk, and pass each other, on the left-hand side of the sidewalk—or the "pavement," as they call it. I never noticed that we Americans walk the way we drive, on the right, but I noticed it in London as I was constantly walking head-on into other pedestrians. The British say "sorry" in instances where we say "excuse me" or "pardon me," but I grew to understand that, at least as it pertained to me, it was an observation. Sometimes, after a sidewalk body slam, men would say, "Sorry, luv," which always thrilled me, as it instantly conjured the image of Michael Caine in *Alfie*.

The London Underground is relatively clean and efficient. The maps are easy to read, and it's cheap, but the word "Underground" is a bit misleading, as it implies that the subway trains run, like most systems, just under the ground. The designers of the London Underground apparently believed that the farther people travel below the earth's mantle, the better. At certain stops it is necessary to go down only two sets of stairs and perhaps an escalator to reach the train platform. But often, when you arrive at your destination, you discover that the train has been slowly descending toward hell, leaving you to scratch your way onto giant cargo elevators, impacted with other denizens of the deep who will join you cheek to cheek on your journey from the center of the earth. I discovered on one of these elevators that I'm claustrophobic, and I had a full-blown panic attack, which involved crying and hyperventilating. Fortunately, the elevator was full of Brits, who, fearing embarrassment—mine or theirs—pretended not to notice.

I was mostly a pedestrian, but when I had to ride, I usually took the bus. New York has tour buses that are replicas of the London double-deckers, but nothing can match riding the real thing. First of all, in New York, nobody would ever allow you to leap onto and off of a moving bus. I love the large platform in the rear from which you must sometimes launch yourself, as it always makes me feel like Lulu from *To Sir, with Love*.

From UCH I would take the number 73 bus to Oxford Street and from there switch to buses going to various destinations. Usually I wouldn't remain at any of these places but would catch another bus returning to Oxford Street. As soon as I hopped onto the bus, I would scramble up the groovy spiral stairs to the top and try to sit as close to the front as possible. If I was lucky enough to get the very front seat, I always felt as if I were on some kind of space-age people mover, careening around corners, eye level with the treetops. For 75p I could sightsee for hours.

ONE DAY EARLY in May, I was told that Jack was scheduled to graduate from Room A of the SCBU to Room B the following day. Room B was for babies who are breathing with little or no supplemental oxygen and therefore need to be monitored slightly less by the nursing staff. It was for healthier babies, babies who were one step closer to being home, and I delightedly hugged the nurse on duty when she gave me the news. For weeks I had walked past Rooms B and C, and envied the families of the babies within. There was a healthier atmosphere about those rooms, less machinery and more baby clothes and toys. Parents held their babies more frequently, and recently, walking past Room B, I'd seen a mother giving her baby a bath. I was thrilled with the news that Jack was doing well enough to move. Twenty-four hours seemed too long to wait.

The next morning I woke up early and ran across the street to the hospital as soon as I was finished submitting to the breast pump. I went straight to Room B, where I found five babies in isolettes, but not one of them was Jack. He was back in his old spot, in Room A.

"I thought Jack was moving to B today," I said to the nurse.

"Yes, I heard something about that, but we have to wait for doctors' rounds. The doctors on duty today must approve the transfer. Don't worry, they'll be coming through in a few hours."

I went back to the nurses' residence and took a shower. It was raining and cold outside, so instead of going to the park, I stayed in my room and wrote some letters. Then, when I figured that the doctors must surely have finished their rounds, I strode back to the hospital and into Room B, where again there was no sign of Jack.

"Doctors are still doing rounds, dear," the nurse in Room B told me. "They'll be finished soon."

I left Room B and stood watching the doctors in Room A. They were examining the baby next to Jack, so I sat down and waited.

Finally they emerged, and Dr. Margaret Snow approached me.

"Mrs. Leary?" she said.

"Yes?"

"I understand that one of the nursing staff told you that Jack might be moving today, but we've decided to keep him on in Room A for another day or two, just to be on the safe side."

"The safe side? What's wrong?"

"Nothing's terribly wrong. He had a few bradys last night, and we don't like his blood-sat reading this morning. Nothing to be terribly alarmed about, but he did have a deep desat or two last night, so we took a blood sample. We'll wait for the results of that before we allow him to move on."

Amazingly, I knew what all of these words meant and was able to counter with, "Wait a minute. Are you worried that he's developing an infection . . . or pulmonary hypertension?"

"We just want to rule out everything. It's probably nothing. A little setback."

"Did you up his theophylline?" I asked.

"We're going to wait for his blood work to come back."

"Hmmm," I said, "I thought clinical trials indicated that theophylline should be used prophylactically in cases—"

For some reason doctors hate being advised on clinical data and neonatal practices by mothers with no medical training. Dr. Snow interrupted me by saying, "Mrs. Leary, I wouldn't worry. I'm sure Jack will be moving to Room B in the next day or two. Let's just wait for those test results." And then she and the resident doctors moved on to examine the babies in Room B.

I spent the rest of the morning sitting mournfully next to Jack's isolette, until Joan Dyer wandered in and said, "Why don't you go for a walk?"

"It's pouring rain, that's why," I replied bitterly.

"Have you ever been to the British Museum? It's only a few minutes' walk from here."

"No," I said.

"Right, well, it's simple really. When you exit the hospital, you walk down Gower Street until you reach Great Russell Street. Turn left, and there it is."

The last thing in the world I wanted to do was visit a museum, but before I knew it, Joan had pushed me out the door of the hospital and sent me off with her umbrella and some cheerful words about Egyptian mummies, Asian artifacts, and the Rosetta Stone.

THE BRITISH MUSEUM'S collections showcase the history of the world's cultures. There is an Africa gallery, America, Britain, Asia, Near East, Pacific galleries, and so on. I didn't pick up a museum guide or look at any maps. I just drifted in and out of the vast exhibition halls on that gloomy afternoon. Around me everywhere were tools, religious icons, and weapons—all evidence of the painstaking efforts of humanity. Staring at these relics now, carefully cataloged and displayed under the pure white gleam of gallery lighting, I was filled with sadness and a sense of futility. The purpose of the museum seemed to be to celebrate man's existence by displaying centuries of our handiwork, but my immediate emotional response was to wonder what all the striving, effort, and elbow grease were for. What was the point of decorating an arrow that was going to break when it was pulled from its prey? Why would a person with a twenty-five-year life expectancy waste time decorating beads?

It was a school day and nearly every exhibit was surrounded by groups of uniformed schoolchildren—lively, rosy-cheeked schoolchildren who breathed effortlessly. Never before had children appeared so robust, so full of health, and as I followed them around the museum I embarked on my usual voyage of doubt: *What if Jack is never able to go to school? What if he always has breathing problems? What if he can't see or hear properly?*

I saw the entrance to the North America gallery and was certain that my mood would be lifted by familiar relics of my own heritage. I expected to find folksy quilts and hand-dipped candles created by people with names like Goody Proctor. Instead the North American wing was filled with the colorful creations of people called Mixtec, Zapotec, and Aztec. People who devoted their time to creating elaborate stone carvings of wind gods, eagle warriors, and jaguars. I learned that these early Native American people were skilled artisans, potters, and metalworkers. I also learned, to my shock and amazement, that, at least as far as the British Museum was concerned, Mexico is in North America. Up until that point, I had honestly believed that North America stopped at the Texas border.

On my way out of the museum, I walked through the Egyptian room. There I was drawn to a rectangular display case in the center of the room that was surrounded by a small crowd. In the case was the almost perfectly preserved body of "Ginger," a five-thousand-year-old man. Ginger had been buried in a shallow sand grave in predynastic Egypt. The lack of bacteria-producing moisture in his desert grave protected him from decay, and so his skin and his ginger-colored hair, even his fingernails and toenails, were perfectly preserved. According to a plaque on Ginger's case, the body had been displayed there in the museum since 1900 and was one of the museum's most popular exhibits. I could see why Ginger drew such a crowd. He was fascinating to look at, and it was hard to walk away. He was curled up, naked, in fetal position, and his flesh was the color of dried mustard. The skin on his head had begun to split open like the seams of a volleyball, and his white skull bone was evident underneath. Beside him lay earthenware jugs and bowls, ceramic beads, and a knife that had been fashioned from a large piece of flint. All these possessions had been carefully placed around him in his grave.

Somebody loved this man, I thought as I looked at these artifacts. My mother had run out and bought Jack a stuffed bunny almost immediately after he was born, and we had placed it in his isolette with a sense of purpose. It almost felt as if there should have been a ceremony for the laying of the bunny with Jack. The bunny was meant to be a comforting presence in what my mother and I thought was a bare and lonely new world. It was about the same size as Jack, and although he was never aware of its presence, whenever we removed it, even for a moment, his isolette seemed to lose all semblance of a home—of a living environment—and we quickly put it back again.

A group of schoolchildren was herded to Ginger's display case by their teacher. The children appeared to be about seven years of age, and they had the glazed, wandering eyes of kids who had shuffled around the museum a few hours too long.

"Is that a real dead person?" one of them asked.

"It's not. It's a chimpanzee," replied another child.

"No, it's a human," the teacher said, and she read them the plaque on Ginger's case. The children jostled for position around the case. There was some shoving, and I saw a little girl angrily stomp the foot of a boy who had accidentally lost his balance and leaned on her for a moment. Two boys were walking around and around the display. Then they stopped and dissolved into hysterical giggles.

"Shhhhh!" admonished the teacher. The boys stopped giggling. One of them pulled the shirtsleeve of the boy next to him and pointed to Ginger. He was pointing at Ginger's anus and deflated testicles, and now all three children were giggling uncontrollably.

"There's nothing funny about that, Robert," said their teacher, but the children couldn't be convinced, and she was forced to wrangle them on to the next exhibit. All the way back to the hospital, I thought about the boys and about poor old Ginger and laughed quietly to myself. When I arrived, I realized

I'd left Joan's umbrella behind, and since it had stopped raining, I went back and retrieved it for her. It was still leaning against Ginger's case, and Ginger still rested within, with his crockery and utensils and his ass bared for all the world to see, as it had been for the past hundred years.

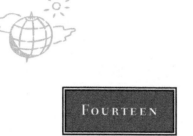

FOURTEEN

I HAD ALWAYS assumed that marriage was an institution created by men. I thought that since men were once biologically unable to prove that a child was theirs, they bound their mates to them by law in an effort to ensure the paternity of their offspring. Now I know different. Marriage was created by women to prevent their men from hightailing it once they got a load of what pregnancy and childbirth can do to the female body and mind. My physical deterioration after Jack's birth was due not only to the usual baby fat and postnatal depression but also to the fact that I couldn't afford to look presentable. Haircuts, eyebrow waxes, and clothing all cost money, and though I had always considered myself a moderately attractive woman, I now came to the sad realization that my looks are purely cosmetic. Without Clinique, I discovered, I am a hag.

I wore my hair short at the time and was already somewhat in need of a haircut when we'd first arrived in London. One day, several weeks after Jack was born, I was walking past a shop window, wearing my usual denim jacket and sunglasses, and, turning to catch a glimpse of my reflection, I was shocked to see Roy Orbison staring back at me.

One of the nurses gave me the name of her hairdresser, whose salon was located within walking distance, near Covent Garden. When I arrived, I was met by George, the owner and sole inhabitant of the salon, who greeted me at the door and shook my hand. He smiled at me, and then his eyes wandered to the sides and top of my head. A cloud came over his face and then he quickly looked back into my eyes and smiled again. It almost seemed as if he was trying not to get caught looking at my hair and that it required the same effort as avoiding looking at a prosthetic limb or a scar. George led me into the salon and had me stand in front of one of the broad, full-length mirrors, and I actually gasped out loud. I hadn't really seen myself in several weeks. I had no mirror in my room, and in the residence bathroom there was only a tiny mirror above the sink. The bathroom in the SCBU had a mirror, but the light in that bathroom never worked, and I could barely make out the shape of my face. George's salon was nothing more than a small room filled with giant mirrors, and under the angry glare of the fluorescent lights, I was now forced to take it all in at once.

The hair was much worse than I'd thought. It had somehow managed to grow out and up instead of down, giving my head the exact shape of an acorn. My face was still puffy from pregnancy, and as a result my eyes were tiny slits. My body, which had always been on the lean side, was now chubby and soft, and my voluminous pants were hiked up over my belly and belted just under my chest, à la Fred Mertz. George must have seen the color drain from my face, as he suddenly steered me away from the mirrors and sent me into a minuscule dressing room to change into a robe. When I emerged, I felt better, since my body was hidden by the robe, and I sat in George's chair and instantly fell asleep.

Sleep was the only positive pregnancy side effect that actually continued after I gave birth to Jack. I'm a lifelong insomniac, and since childhood I've viewed bedtime with a great deal of trepidation, knowing that after everybody else in the house was asleep, I would still be lying there worrying about how tired I was going to be the next day. As soon as I became pregnant, I couldn't get enough sleep. Instead of awakening at my usual 5:00 A.M., I needed the alarm clock to awaken me at seven for work. I would doze on the bus on the way to work, then doze at my desk throughout the day. After work I came home and took a nice long nap, woke up for dinner, then went to bed at nine.

Apparently the hormones and the stress of lactation make new mothers incredibly sleepy, and on my hard dormitory bed, I was still able to lay my head on my pillow and immediately fall asleep. I also, unfortunately, had the tendency to nod off at less appropriate times, as I did that day at George's Salon. When I awoke, I yawned and blinked and tried to look in the mirror, but George turned my chair so that I couldn't see myself. He was frowning and was clearly upset about something. I tried again to look at myself, and George said, "No, no, let me finish." He pushed my hair away from my face, then back over my face. I felt him part my hair on one side, then the other. As I looked at him, it was clear that something had gone terribly wrong, but when I caught his eye, he smiled and said, "Almost ready." Then he took his scissors and trimmed and cut and shaped and slashed, and finally, with a sigh and a tentative smile, he turned me back to the mirror.

Later, back at the hospital, I discovered yet another area in which the social behavior of the British differs from that of Americans. Most Americans, upon seeing a friend or associate with a new hairstyle, will comment favorably upon it, whether it looks nice or not. What's done is done. The person can't usually change her hair back, and the typical American, always determined to bolster the feelings of our fellow Americans, will compliment the new hairstyle no matter how ridiculous it looks. The British have thicker skins than Americans do. Much thicker. I imagine that if you laid the skin of an American out on a table, it would be so thin and delicate that you could see perfectly the surface underneath. The skin of an Englishman or -woman, coarsened by years of bullying and teasing, would, similarly laid out, be thick as cowhide. The British are sincere and see no need to lie to spare the feelings of their friends.

In America responses to my new hairdo might have been something like, "Oh, you have a new haircut. Doesn't that look ni-i-ce!" Or the less hypocritical might simply have said, in an enthusiastic tone, "You got your hair cut!" My new friends at UCH said things like, "Who did that to you?" and "There really ought to be a law. . . ."

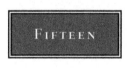
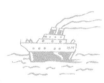

FIFTEEN

ENIS WAS COMING to take us home.

It had been eight long weeks since Jack was born. He had graduated from Room A to Room B. Now he was about to be moved to Room C, which could possibly be his last stop before being released. Jack was gaining weight each day. He breathed on his own and was beginning to nurse. When his weight reached two kilos, approximately four and a half pounds, he would be allowed to go home.

Denis was scheduled to arrive in London on Friday, May 25, and the day before, I went for my usual walk during doctors' rounds. This time, instead of wandering around the park, I went to the local supermarket. Denis and I would be staying at a bed-and-breakfast until Jack's release, and I bought us some snacks for the room and some bottled water and magazines.

I walked back to the hospital, and when I entered Jack's room, I saw Denis standing holding Jack in his arms. He had decided to surprise me by coming a day early. The ward was full of people, but all the fear and loneliness of the past weeks came up and hit me hard when I saw Denis, and I burst into loud, wrenching sobs. The other nurses in the ward grabbed boxes of tissues for themselves, and years later, when I visited the unit, one of the nurses on duty recalled the time I had "sent all the staff into fits of crying" when Denis came back to get us.

THE NEXT DAY Denis and I were discussing our plans for our return to the United States when the chief neonatologist, Dr. Wyatt, overheard us.

"You're not planning to take Jack on an airplane when he's discharged, are you?" he asked.

"Of course we are," I replied.

"I'm afraid Jack's lungs aren't mature enough yet for an airplane flight."

Denis and I both stared at Dr. Wyatt.

"So you're saying we can't take him home?" Denis asked.

"Well, I suppose you could take him home, but you'll have to make some other arrangement besides flying!" Dr. Wyatt said with a chuckle. Then, seeing our astonished stares, he said soberly, "Oxygen levels on aircraft are too unpredictable. *Our* lungs can cope with the rises and falls in oxygen levels, but I'm afraid that it might cause Jack some problems."

Denis and I continued staring at him, desperately searching for a sign that he might be joking.

"I'm terribly sorry. . . . I'm surprised nobody has mentioned this to you before."

THAT NIGHT DENIS and I walked back to the B and B silently. I noticed, when we walked beneath one streetlight, it flickered off and then back on again. I looked up and saw that several of the lights on that block were having problems. They flickered on and off against the night sky, three of them, all in a row.

"Jesus . . . ," I said.

"I know," said Denis.

FOUR YEARS EARLIER, on July 7, 1986, Denis and I were sitting in our Boston apartment reading the Sunday paper, when he said suddenly, "Let's go to the airport. I want to say good-bye to my parents."

Denis's parents were leaving for a monthlong trip to Ireland that evening. It was a trip they had been planning all year.

"We just saw them on the Fourth," I said. "We saw your

whole family on the Fourth of July. Why didn't you say good-bye then?"

"I did," said Denis. "I just want to see them off, that's all."

So we drove to the airport and found Denis's parents and his younger sister, Betsy, in the ticket line. We waited with them and talked about their plans. Then John and Nora and Betsy checked their bags, and we all walked to the security gate together. As we neared the metal detector, we hugged and said our good-byes, and then Denis and I stayed for a moment and watched them disappear into the terminal crowd. Later, on the drive back to Charlestown, Denis said, "I feel bad. I didn't get a chance to shake my dad's hand."

"What?"

"He went through the metal detector before he realized what he was doing, and then Ma was hugging me and everything. I just never got a chance to shake his hand."

Denis usually saw his parents only a few times a year. Although he loved them dearly, he almost never called them on the phone.

"They're only gone a month," I said.

"I know. It just left me with a bad feeling."

"You'll see your dad when they get back," I said, but Denis never saw his father alive again.

Four nights after they arrived in Killarney, John and Nora were at Drum Hall, an Irish club, with John's brother Patrick and his wife, Joan. Patrick and Joan had just arrived, and John went to the bar to buy them a drink. "I still have the five-pound note he was clutching in his hand," Nora says now, when discussing that night. Nora chatted with Joan and Patrick, and then suddenly there was a commotion at the bar. Somebody called out for an ambulance, and Nora and Joan and Patrick ran to find John lying dead next to the bar. He had died instantly of a heart attack.

Denis's mother and Betsy flew back after the Irish wake, and we first spotted them walking through the terminal toward us, huddled together, shocked and gaunt. Nobody had slept in days. None of us could really talk. Nora and Betsy drove back in Denis's brother John's car; Denis, his brother-in-law Neil, and I in another car. Neil had to pull over as we left the airport, and we all sat weeping on the side of the road for a few moments, and then we drove on to Worcester.

It's not convenient to be born or to die overseas. We had to wait a week for John's body to be flown back to Massachusetts. There was a problem obtaining the proper casket in County Kerry, because the casket had to be hermetically sealed for the flight. We spent that week at Denis's parents' house and waited with his mother and brother and sister, his aunts and uncles and cousins. We stayed up until the early-morning hours each night. This was during a heat wave, and we just sat around the living room those nights talking about John and the transportation problems—and also about the lights.

The night that Denis's father died in Ireland, his brother Mick O'Leary stood at his kitchen window and saw lights coming toward him across the field. This caused him great alarm, as there is a family legend that when one of the O'Leary men dies, the death is usually accompanied by strange electrical phenomena. Later, when he learned of John's death, he told his brother and sisters about the lights. That same night, we'd heard, John's brother Patrick had watched a lightbulb from his hall fixture fall right out of its socket and shatter on the floor.

Now that Nora was back, we were having some electrical phenomona Stateside. Nora's power went out one night as we all sat around the living room. Candles were lit, and Neil was just making his way down to the cellar to have a look at the circuit breaker when the power came back on. "It's the heat wave," somebody said. "There's a power shortage." And somebody else said, "It's John. He's showing us he's here, with us now."

There were light stories all week. A family friend left the Learys', and when he arrived home, his porch light was flickering on and off. People arrived home to find lights on that they were sure they'd left off. I have to say that at the time I had some doubt about some of these stories. They probably didn't remember that they'd left the light on, I thought. Lights flicker.

Ann Marie and Neil Coleman, Denis's sister and brother-in-law, had recently bought their first home. On the front lawn was an old gaslight that had never worked since they'd had the house. John had come over to have a look at the light just before he left for Ireland. "I'll fix it when we get back from Ireland," he'd promised Ann Marie. The week that we waited for John's body, Ann stayed at her mother's. Finally she needed some clothes for the funeral, so she went home, and though it was the middle of the day, the gaslight was lit, and it worked from that point on.

Over the years, when we have family get-togethers, something always happens. A couple will announce they're pregnant and the chandelier above will suddenly dim for a moment—or some of us will think it dimmed. On Christmas Eve, when everybody is finally under one roof, somebody will go to switch on a light and the bulb will blow. Then everybody laughs and blames Dad, except Nora, the cynic, who says, "That was an old lightbulb. It just burned out." Now, walking down this historic street in a once foreign city, the flickering streetlights had a soothing, reassuring effect, and left us with the feeling you only receive from a loving parent—the feeling that we were at home and that we were being cared for.

IT WAS EARLY June, and we needed a flat to rent for the entire summer. Unfortunately, we discovered upon visiting several estate agents that short-term summer rentals in London are outrageously expensive, meant to be leased for one or two weeks at a time by tourists on holiday.

"I never envisioned this," I said to Denis one afternoon after being laughed at by an agent when we told him what we were able to pay for a rental. "I just somehow assumed that when we had our first baby, we wouldn't be homeless."

We were, in fact, entirely homeless. We were so broke with

our London expenses that we couldn't afford the rent on our Boston apartment. We had to let it go. It was the home where we had conceived our child, where I had wandered about dreamily for five months, thinking, *This is where I'll feed the baby,* and *I'll put the baby's bassinet here in the mornings,* and *I'd better fix that exposed electrical outlet before the baby comes.* Denis had packed up our things in a haphazard fashion one day and moved them into my mother's garage, leaving behind the baby's room littered with remains of our former life. When we returned to the States, the plan was that I would stay at my mother's house for a few weeks while Denis looked for an apartment in New York and earned enough money to put down a deposit.

The hospital social worker had given me a list of charitable organizations that provided emergency housing, and I was just about to start on this list when Jo called with the exciting news that she had found us a flat. Somehow Jo's investigative genius had led her to a one-bedroom flat in Islington. Its tenant was an American man who had suddenly learned that he needed to return to California for a few months. He would sublet us his place at the same rental rate that he had been paying. This we could afford, because Denis now had a regular source of income in the UK. Not long after Denis's initial appearance on *Live from Paramount City,* he had met John Thoday of Avalon Entertainment. John managed several successful British comedians, and he began booking Denis in comedy clubs in and around London.

*   *   *

IN THE SCBU at University College Hospital are two parents' rooms. These are rooms where parents can sit and read or use breast pumps in relative privacy. When a baby is ready to be discharged from the hospital, the rooms are used as sleeping-in rooms for the parents and the soon-to-be-released infant. I don't know if such a setup exists in American hospitals, but it was a wonderful way to make the transition from being an institutionalized pseudofamily to being a real family. Denis and Jack and I slept in this room for two nights. Denis and I bathed Jack, I nursed him, we dressed him and put him to bed, all in the safety of the hospital where Jack had lived his entire life. If his color changed for an instant, we sprinted down the hall with him in our arms, just to have a resident doctor or nurse reassure us that he was fine. We felt like children playing house in a larger house that was run by grown-ups, and I personally would have been happy to keep on with this arrangement until Jack's eighteenth birthday. The initial resentment I'd felt toward the hospital staff for usurping my role as a parent had been replaced by utter dependence. Despite the many weeks of hoping and praying for the day when Jack would be well enough to go home, now that the time had arrived, I was terrified.

Before babies are discharged from the SCBU, they must be examined by a physician, so Denis and I passed Jack's final morning in the hospital saying our emotional good-byes to the other parents and to the staff. Finally it was time for Jack to be examined by a Dr. Singh, whom we had not met before. He declared Jack healthy enough to go home and wished us luck. Then he said to me, "You must try very hard to leave this experience behind you now."

"Okay," I said vacantly, as I swaddled Jack tightly in a blanket. When I lifted him from the table, I checked his cheeks for color and quickly felt his pulse, just to make certain that the examination wasn't too taxing. Then I pulled a wool hat over his head and tucked him into the carry pouch that was strapped across my chest.

"This is exactly what I'm talking about," said Dr. Singh. "We're having a heat wave. You don't need to bundle the baby so."

"Do you think he's too hot?" I asked in a panic.

"Yes. I think, maybe."

I had read that overheating was considered a likely cause of crib death, and although I was not aware of a baby's ever succumbing to crib death outside a crib, it seemed altogether likely that it could happen. I frantically pulled off the hat and began unwrapping Jack's many layers.

"I'm saying this for his sake more than yours," said Dr. Singh. "I've seen it happen that these babies grow up into children who are too protected—too precious—and it isn't healthy for them, physically or emotionally. He's fine now. Try to forget that he was premature, and treat him like any other newborn."

I know that Dr. Singh was right. It's always better not to make a child too precious, but the problem is that children *are* just so unspeakably precious, all of them, and especially the uncertain, precarious ones like Jack. I wondered if Dr. Singh actually expected any parent to be able to follow his advice after the ordeal of the Special Care Baby Unit. Just two weeks earlier, Jack had been regularly setting off his apnea alarm because he still couldn't always remember to breathe, but now I was supposed to put him to bed each night without a second thought.

Normally the birth of one's first child is, I think, supposed to be life-affirming, but the circumstances surrounding Jack's arrival had shaken loose my tentative grasp of faith in God and humanity. I had seen a baby born with missing limbs and babies with swollen, bleeding brains. I saw a newborn girl who had been born with her intestines on the outside of her body. I saw babies born to drug addicts, and I saw a man say to his wife, about a very sick premature black baby, "Look at the wee monkey!" and I watched them both snort with laughter. I saw a baby born weighing less than a pound, who existed for only a few days, long enough to taunt the parents with a glimpse of what might have been, and then he was gone forever. Now, for Jack's own good, I was supposed to act as if it all had never happened.

THIS IS IT, Jack . . . you're free!" exclaimed Denis as we carried him out of the hospital for his first breath of outside air. Jack slept in his pouch, with his cheek against my chest. Denis and I walked carefully along the sidewalk for a few feet, and then I stopped.

"He's not breathing," I said.

"Let me see," said Denis, peering into Jack's face. Then he said frantically, "Let's go back!"

We turned and, hearts pounding, started walking rapidly back toward the hospital doors. Then I saw Jack move his head, and he gave a little cry.

"I think he's okay," I said, grabbing Denis's arm.

"Do you think he's breathing?" asked Denis.

"Well, I think you can't cry without breathing. Look . . . he's trying to suck his thumb. He's fine," I said, and then we turned our backs on the hospital for good.

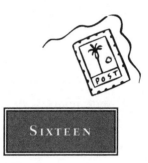

Sixteen

E TOOK A taxi to our new lodgings on Thornhill
Road in Islington, where we were met by Caroline, the
owner of the house. Jo had told me that Caroline was the
mother of five and a grandmother, but the woman who opened
the door with a warm smile was younger looking than I had
anticipated. She wore hip, baggy trousers and Birkenstocks,
and her graying hair was caught up in a sloppy ponytail.

"There he is," she said, nodding at Jack. "Your friend Jo told
me the baby is two months old but still has a month before he's
due to be born. I've been quite curious to have a look at him."

I turned so that Caroline could see Jack's sleeping face.

"Hmmm," she said. "Well, he's got all his bits and pieces,
doesn't he? I'm quite amazed, really. I wasn't sure what to

expect when your friend told me about what had happened. Marvelous what medical science can do today!"

"Oh . . . thank you," I said. I was certain that Caroline had complimented Jack somehow.

Caroline showed us our flat on the third floor. There was a small kitchen with a table and two chairs set against a window that looked down upon lovely Thornhill Road. Although there was no dishwasher, there was a machine that both washed and dried clothing. This machine didn't know it, but it was about to start running twenty-four hours a day for the next several months. Next to the kitchen was a living room with a television and a well-stocked bookcase. And across from the living room were a bedroom and a bathroom. Caroline explained how everything worked and told us to knock on the door of her first-floor flat if we needed anything. Then she left us, and there we stood, for the first time alone together—a family.

That afternoon I wandered around our new home and visualized my daily routine. At seven in the morning, the time I usually went to the SCBU to nurse Jack, he would awaken, I imagined, so I would put a fresh diaper on him, nurse him, and then set him in his little basket to sleep while I showered and then enjoyed my own breakfast. At eleven I would nurse Jack again, then put him into the "pram" that Jo had loaned me, and we would take our morning stroll around the neighborhood. This would allow Denis time to work on writing his show. Arriving back at the house around noon, I would carry the pram up to the flat and leave the sleeping Jack in it while I ate lunch and had a nap. Then, in the afternoons, I would do the laundry and tidy up the flat. Later I would make dinner for Denis and me, and the three of us would take an evening stroll around the neighborhood before we tucked Jack into bed for the night at seven-thirty. Then, in the evenings, I would read or watch TV while Denis went to work.

During the first days and weeks after Jack's birth, I had been amazed at my heightened energy level. Jo commented on it frequently. After Florence's birth, she told me, she was absolutely "knackered" for months. She never could have done all the running around that I was doing, she said. At the time I just assumed I was of heartier stock than the average Brit. Sure, the English have a scholarly advantage over the average American, I thought, but in a match of strength—a rasslin' match, for example—you'd always want your money on the American. Bolstered by hormones, I met life with a personally unprecedented gusto. I'd never had major surgery before and was pleased to discover that my recuperative powers were so superior. Within days of Jack's birth, I was skipping down the stairs to the SCBU two at a time, frantic to see my baby. I ate like a horse, raced back and forth between the hospital and the nurses' home and the park many times a day, and at night I laid my head upon the pillow and instantly fell into a deep and restorative sleep. I had no idea that what makes new mothers so tired—so dreadfully, horribly tired—is not the giving birth but the actual *taking care of* the baby.

During those first weeks on Thornhill Road, my day began

not at seven, as I had planned, but rather at around one in the morning. I kept Jack's basket on a large ottoman at the foot of our bed, and every hour or so, he would awaken. His first little cry would cause me to sit bolt upright in bed, and within a microsecond I had scrambled on all fours down to the end of the bed to scoop him up. Then I would carry him back to my pillow. This always required me to move across the bed supported by both knees and one knuckle, the other arm clutching Jack, mama-baboon style, against my chest. Propped up against my pillows, I would nurse Jack drowsily but not allow myself to doze off for fear that Denis or I might crush him in our sleep. I would nurse Jack back to sleep, and then I would crawl back to the end of the bed to place him in his basket. I would go back to sleep and would be awakened again at two, then at three, and every hour after that each night.

All the eating and bathing and sleeping in that flat was done by Jack, and he did all these things several times each hour. All the strolls around the neighborhood and house tidying that I had imagined were pipe dreams. Most days I would find myself still dressed in my nightgown at five in the afternoon. My hair would be plastered to my head, and I would be nursing Jack and shoveling handfuls of meat into my mouth. (I was on a ham bender and had decided that the bread-placement part of making the sandwich was simply too exhausting.) Denis would usually stagger into the room, having just woken up from a nap, and, hungrily eyeing the meat, he'd make a move for it. My mouth too full to speak, I'd issue a throaty growl, and he'd retreat into the kitchen to forage for himself. We both were testing the human capacity for sleeplessness, and our marriage had turned into a Darwinian experiment of sorts.

IN ENGLAND, IF a woman has a normal delivery that produces a healthy child, she and the baby are usually sent home within twenty-four hours. Once she arrives home, the local health authority is notified of the birth, and for the next ten days, if necessary, every day a midwife visits the home to check on the health of the mother and child. After ten days the midwife hands the family's case over to a health visitor, who is a registered nurse. British citizens are required to allow the health visitor to come at least once, to assess the family's living conditions and to ensure that parents and baby are coping well. When I first heard about this home visiting, I thought it was wonderful. No wonder British babies have a higher survival rate than American babies do during their first year, I thought, having recently read this statistic. And how nice for the parents not to have to take the baby out to a germy doctor's office during those first weeks, if something is wrong.

In fact, the health visitor seemed to be viewed by most of the English people I knew as a mixed blessing. It *is* comforting to have a professional come into your home to offer assistance, but, in fact, mandatory health visiting began as an effort to control epidemics in London slums. Because the practice had its origins as a sanitary rather than a strictly medical concern, people still partially view it as the government's snooping into families' lives. Jo had told me that when she was a little girl, the health visitor tended to show up unannounced, which would cause her mother to shriek, "The bloody health visitor! Quick, clear up!" Jo said that health visitors have an uncanny knack for showing up "just when the mum has lost her temper and clipped her oldest child on the ear," and so their visits were usually viewed with some trepidation, which was exactly how I viewed the impending visit of our health visitor.

Before we were released from the hospital, we had to register with the local council of Islington. Within a week of our arrival, the health visitor phoned to say that she'd like to "call round" the next morning. I hung up the phone and burst into tears. *The jig is up,* I thought. The British government is sending a health worker to assess our abilities as parents and, seeing how woefully incapable we are, will remove Jack and place him in a foster home, with qualified, experienced parents. I looked around the flat and had no idea where to begin cleaning. Every vertical surface, every chair back, radiator, door, and hanger was draped with drying laundry—all of it Jack's. Jack's personal habits, which involved milk spewing from his mouth after every feeding, and other fluids incessantly leaking from below, required a complete change of clothing nearly every hour. The machine that was supposed to wash and dry the clothes just washed and tossed them for what seemed like hours. When the drying cycle was finished, the clothes came out soaking wet and had to be hung to dry. The sink was filled with dirty dishes. Our bedroom was a disaster. We had never found the right time to unpack our clothing, so we'd just started pulling things out of our suitcases as we needed them and then throwing them wherever we felt like it before passing out in bed each night. Denis had been booked into a club hours from London the night before and had arrived home in the early morning, but I had no pity. I bullied him out of bed, and he tried to help me get the place in order, but it was no use. Every time we folded something of Jack's, it needed to be unfolded and worn. The dirty jammies and onesies and bibs just kept coming. The kitchen washing machine was no match for our four-pound son's wardrobe. I finally decided that if we at least cleaned the kitchen and bathroom, we couldn't be brought up on charges, so we scrubbed and cleaned, and then Denis brought home fish and chips for dinner.

The next morning the health visitor arrived, as she had announced, at ten o'clock. She buzzed us on the intercom, and I buzzed her in, against my better judgment. Denis had worked late again the night before and had awoken during most of Jack's nighttime feedings. Now he couldn't be roused. I envisioned the health visitor as a hefty, highly starched matron along the lines of the SCBU's Miss Borthwick, who would no doubt cast a disapproving eye about our flat and, seeing Denis passed out in bed, demand that he produce a urine specimen right before her eyes for a drug test.

I heard a sharp knock on the door, and when I opened it, with Jack draped over my shoulder, I met one of the cheeriest, prettiest girls I had ever encountered in England. She wore smart, casual street clothes, not the matron's uniform that I'd imagined, and she grabbed my free hand and shook it.

"I'm Jane Williams," she said. "What a lovely flat."

Jane followed me into the sitting room, and I was at a bit of a loss as to what to do next.

"Would you like something to drink?" I asked.

"I'd love a cup of tea, actually," replied Jane.

Of course, why hadn't I thought of that? The English always offer tea to visitors.

"Okay," I said. "Let's just go into the kitchen."

As soon as I started to fill the teakettle, Jack woke up and began crying, and I started to get flustered, bouncing him in one arm and trying to turn on the stove with the other.

"I'll hold him for you, if you'd like," offered Jane, and I gratefully handed him over.

By the time we finished our tea I felt as if we were old friends. Jack lay draped across Jane's lap, facedown, like a sack of potatoes, sleeping peacefully. Jane told me that many babies cry and fuss because their tummies hurt, and this position helps them. When I told her about the constant feeding and spitting up, she suggested that instead of feeding him every time he fussed, I should try putting him in this position. She said his little tummy was probably just too full. She also said that, in her opinion, always comforting babies with food might later cause eating disorders, since the child learns that food is not only nourishment but an emotional crutch.

"That's just a theory of mine," she said. "Try cuddling him, and then, if he still whinges, feed him."

"Well, okay," I said, "but I don't know if you've ever cared for a baby who was as premature as Jack. He only weighed about two pounds when he was born, and—"

"Oh, yes," said Jane. "I know. I've seen all his records. There's another baby on my watch who was less than two pounds when he was born. Lives not far from here, really. He's doing remarkably well. I've had quite a few SCBU graduates the past few years," she added with a reassuring smile, and then I bombarded her with all the fears, doubts, and concerns I had encountered during our first week at home, and Jane answered all my questions with reassuring, educated responses.

"Look, he's waking up," said Jane as Jack let out a little bleat. She turned him over and looked into his face. "He's gorgeous!" she exclaimed, and my heart swelled with pride.

"Are you familiar with infant massage?" asked Jane.

"Not exactly," I replied.

"Well, last summer I took a course in Sweden in massage therapy, and I'm really fascinated by it. So when I returned to London, I began to learn infant-massage techniques. I'd be happy to teach you some methods that might be beneficial to Jack. Massage is excellent for the respiratory and circulatory systems."

Jane hadn't inspected my bathroom or asked where my husband was hiding himself. Instead she was showing me the exact spot on Jack's tiny little foot where a pressure point existed that, when gently massaged, would relieve colicky symptoms. She showed me how to work my fingers in small circles all over his back and up and down his legs.

"There's a theory that massage might help prevent the developmental delays that many preemies experience. I don't know that it's been scientifically proven yet, but it can't hurt. Look how he's enjoying this," Jane said, "and it actually has been proven that massage helps strengthen the immune system." Jane was obviously a massage nut, and I felt like she'd been sent from heaven above. Then, before I knew it, it was time for her to leave.

"So soon?" I asked, trying to conceal the desperation in my voice.

"Yeah, I've two more calls before lunch."

"When can you come back?" I asked, making an effort not to whine.

"I shouldn't think you'll need me back. You're doing a great job," Jane said. "You're so relaxed! Most first-time mums in your position are total wrecks. You Americans are so easygoing! Here's my card. If you have any questions at any time, feel free to phone me." Then Jane was gone, and I was left holding my blissful, utterly massaged baby boy.

SEVENTEEN

*D*ENIS AND I met Betty, our eighty-five-year-old neighbor, during our first week in the house on Thornhill Road. We were sitting in the back garden with Jack when she approached, shuffling toward us in a faded housedress, bent so far forward at the waist that at first I thought she was looking for something on the ground. When she finally reached the bench where we sat, she tilted her head up, allowing a view of one bewhiskered ear, one eye, and half of a near-toothless smile, and said, giggling into her hand, "'Ave you seen me pussy?"

Denis and I, both certain that we were in the company of a woman in an advanced state of senility, with exhibitionism on her decaying mind, cried out, "NO!" and "PLEASE, NO!" and

"SHOULDN'T YOU BE INDOORS ON SUCH A HOT DAY?" shielding our eyes and ducking our heads.

"'E's rather old," replied Betty. "Almost twenty, me Timmy is, but still 'e likes to wander. All I 'ave in this world is me pussycat."

"Oh," I said. "How long has he been missing? Maybe we can help you find him."

"True, 'tis hot. Still, I like to take in a little sun of an afternoon," Betty said, her eye now cast on the bench where we sat.

Denis sprang to his feet. "Sit down! I have some phone calls to make," and Denis made his escape, with lightning speed, into the house.

Jack was asleep in my arms, and I moved over on the bench to make room for Betty, who sat down gratefully. It was now clear that she suffered from an advanced case of osteoporosis, as she retained the bent, leaning conformation even while seated. Betty told me, with her face tilted up in my direction, that she lived on the second floor and, with very little encouragement from me, began sharing her life story, which I won't detail on these pages except for the amazing fact that Betty had lived in that same house on Thornhill Road most of her adult life. When she began to describe the night that the neighborhood was bombed during the Blitz, I pumped her for details, but as soon as she got to the part where the air-raid sirens sounded, she strayed into an account of the duplicitous behavior of a former housemate named Lily. In those days, according to Betty, the house's denizens were all female lodgers, and Betty told me that afternoon, and over the course of many afternoons in that garden in the weeks to come, about her very close friendship with Lily. From what I could gather, Betty was bitterly jealous of Lily's friendship with another resident of the house, named Nell.

"Lily always liked a nice 'ot cuppa, even of a steamy summer afternoon, but that day I made the tea, and Lily announced that she and *Nell*"—Betty always spit out Nell's name with a look of extreme distaste—"already 'ad their tea *iced,* thank you very much, in *Nell's* room."

Though I tried, I never did get the fine details about the German bombers, but I did get a pretty clear picture of the level of sexual tension that had existed in the house, which ultimately led me to the conclusion that Betty and several other wartime lodgers might have been frustrated lesbians. Which brings me to another point. I've never been great at determining the sexuality of others, but in England I was totally lost in this regard. Denis and I had become friends with several British comedians by then, and upon first meeting them, I thought each and every one was gay. This also held true for most of the hospital staff at University College Hospital and the majority of parents. In America, if a man is lean, relatively fashion-conscious, particularly witty, and enjoys the company of women, it's a pretty safe bet he's gay. Similarly, in America one might assume that a somewhat masculine woman who is hairy, clueless about fashion, and particularly enjoys the company of other women is a lesbian. In England people of both sexes, whether gay or not, find the company of women enjoyable, and to further confuse things, men know an awful lot about fashion and women seem to know a lot about everything except for fashion.

By the time we moved to Thornhill Road, I doubted my initial hunch that all our neighbors were gay. Sure, Robert and Brian, who had the other third-floor flat, were both incredibly sweet and hilariously funny, and Brian referred to Robert as "luv," but based on what I had seen of heterosexual male behavior in Britain, this meant nothing. Also, Caroline, the landlord, wore Birkenstocks with socks almost every day, but I had met several mothers at the hospital who did so as well.

"If I didn't know better," I said to Denis after spotting Caroline in the garden French-kissing her friend Sandra not long after we had moved in, "I'd think everybody in this house was gay except for us."

"Everybody in this house *is* gay except for us, and . . . and, I suppose, Timmy," replied Denis, who has always had pitch-perfect gay/straight cognizance. Eventually everybody in that house let us know that they were in fact gay, except Betty and Timmy, and they were all very kind to us and became very fond of Jack—except for Timmy, who, I was convinced, was plotting the baby's murder from the day we first set foot through the door.

I have always been an animal lover. As a child I planned to be a veterinarian when I grew up. A veterinarian who raised dogs and horses, lived on a cattle ranch, and was married to a cowboy. As I matured, I slowly saw the insanity of my dream—you have to get good grades to go to vet school, and there are no cowboys in the Boston area—but I retained my love for animals until Jack was born. Then I began to see most four-legged creatures as predators.

That summer there had been a series of horrible dog attacks in the London area that made the news. In London, as in most American cities, pit bull terriers and rottweilers had become trendy among gang members. The pit bulls were used in dog fights and as props for their owners to look cool and menacing walking down the street. Kids began breeding these dogs indiscriminately in housing projects and tenements and were producing some vicious dogs who began attacking neighbors, children, and other pets. In a London park, a man walking home from work was attacked by a couple of pit bulls and savaged so badly that there was really nothing left of his face. Each morning I read the tabloid accounts of these maulings while sitting in the park near our flat and I clutched Jack protectively against my chest. Denis read the same accounts and used them for material in his stand-up routine. Before Jack, I was always making friends with strange dogs in parks, but now, even if the dog was being walked past on a leash, even if it was a Labrador or a cocker spaniel, I veered off the path to make room for it, longing for a large stick or a gun to use as a defensive weapon.

I decided that first summer of motherhood that even more terrifying than dogs were cats. I had read in one of my British baby-care books that the baby should have plenty of fresh air and that although it's a good idea to allow the baby to nap in his pram in the garden, the pram must be covered with a protective mesh or screen, to keep cats off. Cats, I learned, will sometimes jump into the pram. Then, always looking for a warm spot to lie down, the cat will choose the baby's face and smother it to death. Somehow this became inflated in my paranoid mind, and I imagined that Timmy lay in wait for us each afternoon—keeping an eye out for that moment when my back was turned—and then he would pounce into Jack's pram to suck the very life breath out of his tiny form. I worried that Timmy might sneak into the flat somehow and make his way into Jack's basket while he was sleeping. I grew to hate Timmy. Sometimes I would encounter him on the stairs, grooming himself, a stiff, arthritic leg extended over his head, his wizened face pausing for a moment to glower at me, before returning to the licking of his matted tail, and I would fix him with a menacing stare. Sometimes I would lift my shoe in his direction, just to give him an idea of how easy it would be for me to send him sailing, head over matted tail, down the staircase. I'm ashamed to say now that one afternoon as he sat on the garden fence eyeballing Jack's pram with a twitching tail, I plotted his demise. *Nobody'll ever trace the poison back to me,* I thought. A cat like Timmy must have a lot of enemies. Or maybe a fall from a window. "I saw him try to jump up onto the windowsill," I would tell the detective, "but he was unable to catch himself. Poor kitty."

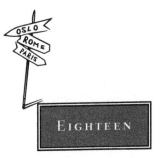

Eighteen

ORMALLY AN INFANT receives his first inoculations against diphtheria, tetanus, pertussis, and polio when he's eight weeks old. When Jack was eight weeks old, he was just being discharged from the hospital and still wasn't due to be born for another month. The doctors at UCH had told me that he was scheduled for the vaccinations anyway. They said that the National Health Service recommends that preemies receive immunizations on the same schedule following their birth dates as full-term babies. Later, when Jane the health visitor came, she also urged me to schedule the vaccinations at the local clinic as soon as possible. By this time I had done some research. I knew that vaccinations for preemies were somewhat controversial. Immunizations stress the immune system, and a preemie's immune system is already stressed. I had also read an article theorizing that some SIDS cases seemed to be related to vaccinations. When your baby spends his first two months constantly forgetting to breathe, sudden infant death syndrome becomes a fixation. I don't think an hour went by in those early months that SIDS didn't cross my mind. Jack was already at risk, so the idea of injecting him with germs that might make him even more at risk made me wild with fear, and I followed Denis around for days badgering him about the situation.

"Suppose he gets sick from the vaccination and dies, simply because we made the reckless decision to have him vaccinated," I said the minute Denis woke up one morning.

"What do the doctors say?" Denis asked wearily.

"The *doctors!*" I replied. "The *doctors* in this country work for the government. They make decisions based on what is healthiest for the masses. They can't make exceptions for individual cases like ours."

"I don't know how many times I have to say this," Denis said, "but you're not a doctor, and these 'doctors of the masses' have done fine by Jack so far. If we were home, wouldn't you have him vaccinated? Wouldn't we have to?"

"I don't know!" I cried.

"Well, what if we don't vaccinate him and he catches . . . whatever . . ."

"Diphtheria, whooping cough!"

"Whatever," said Denis impatiently. "How could we live with ourselves then?"

"Well, I've already thought of that and it really shouldn't be too difficult to avoid contact with other people until Jack's a little older. I could stop taking him to the grocery store and on the bus—"

"Yeah, that's good because all the diphtheria victims travel by bus," Denis said. "I think you should do what the doctors suggest."

The next day I received a phone call from Jane the health visitor, telling me that I should bring Jack to the local clinic the following Wednesday, July 3, for his vaccinations.

"That's funny," I said, "July third was Jack's original due date. I feel like I've been a mother forever, and he's not even supposed to be born yet. He's so tiny. I don't know. . . ."

"Just go and get it over with," said Jane. "They'll weigh him and everything, and you'll feel more at ease when it's over. You'll be flying home with him before long, and you don't want him on an international flight with all those germs."

"All right, all right," I said, and the next Wednesday I took Jack to the local clinic.

All English councils have a community health clinic with one or more GPs, or general practitioners. The GP performs all duties that most Americans now entrust to specialists like obstetricians, pediatricians, gynecologists, and internists. The GP, like the old-fashioned American country doctor, looks after all the babies and old men and pregnant women in his council, and I imagined that my local GP would be a fatherly Marcus Welby type. I thought it likely that when I arrived at the clinic, a sweet, plump nurse would welcome me into an oak-paneled office, where I would find the doctor seated at an antique desk. He would invite me to sit hearthside in an overstuffed chair and would ask me all about Jack's health and mine. Then he would administer the vaccinations so gently that Jack would sleep through the whole thing, and when it was all over, he would reassure me with a warm embrace and send me on my way.

I arrived at the clinic at ten o'clock on Wednesday, just as Jane had instructed, and when I walked through the front door, I found myself in a long, narrow hallway. The hallway was lined on both sides with benches that were occupied with women holding babies. It was a rare, bright London morning that I had left outside, and I had trouble adjusting my eyes to the dimness in this windowless, antiseptic space. The other women were reading or breast-feeding and chatting quietly with one another. Some had older children with them, and a few were accompanied by their husbands. I walked along the benches until I came upon a window with a door next to it. Behind the window was a nurse with a clipboard. I told her Jack's name, and she checked it off a long list and asked me to have a seat. I found a spot on the bench and sat down. Jack, missing the lull of my pace, awoke. I removed him from his pouch and put him to my breast, and I sat with the other mothers and babies and waited. I realized that all these women were here to have their babies vaccinated, and all the babies, except for Jack, appeared to be about two months old. In their company Jack looked like the world's tiniest eighty-year-old. He still hadn't acquired the plump baby features that would later cause Caroline, our landlord, to comment that Jack seemed to be growing younger by the day. He had a worried, age-worn look, and I was aware of it only now that I was surrounded by these fleshy full-term babies.

The woman seated next to me was turned slightly away, as she was talking with her neighbor, and her baby was held against her shoulder, facing me. I looked at the baby, and he looked back at me, but he was so close that he could take in only a little of me at a time. First the baby stared seriously at my chin, then looked right at my nose. Then, wobble-headed, he moved his eyes around my face, and when they finally settled on my own eyes, the baby's face froze for a moment in surprise, and then it lit up with a bright smile of recognition. The baby knew me for what I was, and I smiled back almost involuntarily. I felt obliged to confirm for him our human kinship, and we remained for a moment, eyes locked and smiling. Then he bit his mother's neck, and she lowered him onto her lap.

We waited for what seemed like hours. The clinic vaccinates babies only once or twice a month, I discovered. I sat there and fretted about the baby with the runny nose on my left and the close air in the waiting hall, and I recalled a chapter in one of my baby books that had warned of the dangers of vaccinating a sick baby. What if Jack contracted whatever vile infection the baby next to me carried and then was vaccinated at exactly the same time? Would he survive? Perhaps a bigger baby stood a chance, I thought, but Jack was so little. . . .

Finally Jack's name was called, and I carried him into the

examination room. Marcus Welby wasn't there. Just a nurse who asked me to undress Jack and place him on a baby scale. He was a whopping six pounds, nine ounces, and I remembered suddenly that today was Jack's due date—the date he was meant to be born—and I wondered what his real birth weight would have been if he had gone to term. Would he have weighed more or less? I wondered, and as the nurse swabbed Jack's tiny bicep, the smell of rubbing alcohol brought me back to the SCBU and the alarms and tubes and babies made of skin and bones and little else. I watched the needle approach Jack's arm. The syringe was loaded with manufactured disease that, I hoped, would ward off the more serious biological plagues of our world, and when the needle pierced his skin—his clean, delicate baby skin—I gasped aloud, then burst into tears.

"I'm sorry," I muttered.

"Don't worry," said the nurse. "It's not the first time I've made the mum cry louder than the baby. He must be your firstborn."

"He is," I sobbed, and then I carried Jack out of the clinic. We went home and found Denis working in the kitchen. He was writing notes for his act, and when I walked in, I was still teary-eyed. I told Denis about the clinic and the vaccinations. I already felt that Jack seemed somehow weaker, even though he was sound asleep.

"He just doesn't seem the same," I said.

"Give him to me."

I lifted Jack out of his pouch and handed him over. Jack blinked and made a little crying noise and then nodded back off to sleep. Denis held him up and looked him over carefully. He gazed at his face, and then he sniffed his head and kissed his hair.

"He's fine," Denis declared. "There's nothing wrong with him." Then Denis handed him back to me, and I saw that he really was fine, and I made a silent vow to be like Denis and never read another book or article about pediatrics or neonatology.

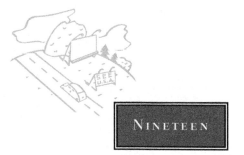

NINETEEN

BEFORE JACK WAS born, I had never considered myself particularly patriotic, but now just the word "America" made me weak with longing. I was tired of being an obliging guest in a foreign city, tired of laughing at anti-American jokes, and tired of the unattractive aspect of my personality that I hadn't had a chance to discover before being trapped in a foreign country: It turns out that I'm an inveterate turncoat. It frightens me sometimes to think how hasty I am to join ranks with the other side. Not only did I try to behave as much like a Brit as I possibly could that long summer, but I would usually agree with anyone who had a negative, sarcastic word about the United States. For example, a doctor taking a break outside the unit one day, while Jack was still in the hospital, described to me a film he had seen the night before. The film was *The Hunt for Red October.*

"Typical Hollywood tripe," he said.

I said, "Yes, those *Hollywood* films, they just . . . suck."

"Mind you, you know what you're getting when you put your six pounds down for an American film. You know you're going to walk out all excited about the special effects and the action scenes, but later you'll realize that the film was not only mind-numbingly stupid, but the actors don't know the first thing about acting."

"I know." And then I said, "I'm embarrassed to be an American when I see films like *The Hunt for Red October.* I really am. Give me a good Merchant-Ivory film any day."

I had actually just seen *The Hunt for Red October.* I had splurged the previous week and walked down to the Empire Cinema in Leicester Square, and I can easily count it as one of the top five most exciting experiences of my life.

Although the multiplex is slowly taking over, there are several grand cinemas left in London, and the Empire is one of them. When you arrive at the box office, the ticket seller provides you with a seating chart and you can choose your seats, just like at a theater box office. Then you make your way into a velvet-draped lobby and find a concession stand that offers both salted and sugared popcorn, a wide array of other snacks, and beer and wine. I hadn't been out at night in such a long time that I was literally dazzled by the sheer thrill of leaving the dark street and entering such a bright, lively environment. I bought a popcorn and a Coke and climbed the stairs to the balcony seats I had chosen. I was in the first row of the balcony, in my mind the most coveted seats in any theater, and I settled in with my snacks just in time for the commercials and trailers. I never knew advertising could be so entertaining! And then the film began, with a panoramic shot of the sea, and when a submarine surfaced, it sent forth a Dolby-enhanced spray of surf that seemed so real I actually ducked. I felt like an Aboriginal bushman being shown his first movie, and my heart raced, and I realized that my cheeks were sore from smiling. Now, discussing the dismal state of American films with a British doctor, however, I shook my head in disgust at the mere mention of the film.

I realize now how fortunate I am that I never crossed paths with a Hare Krishna or a Moonie—I'm such a ready convert. I always knew that Patty Hearst was innocent. Put in her position, I never could have held out as long as she did. Within minutes of being captured by the Symbionese Liberation Army, I would have said, "Hand me that gun, gorgeous," to the creepy ringleader, and that would have been me posing in the bank with a jaunty beret.

It wasn't until Denis and I were living together in Islington that I began to feel I could behave like an American—and behave like Americans we did. Every Thursday was trash-collection day on Thornhill Road, and all the other tenants of that house would carry their week's supply of garbage down to the road. They would need to make only one trip, as their week's refuse could fit into a bag so small it looked as if it were carrying a child's lunch. Our week's supply of garbage was contained in about twenty industrial-size garbage bags, and on Thursdays we had to devote the better part of the afternoon to its removal. We would put Jack down for a nap and begin the countless trips up and down the stairs until we had removed the last bag and the road in front of the house looked as though it had been barricaded against a nuclear assault. Sometimes we would catch a glimpse of Caroline staring out her window at us, and I would say, "This is embarrassing. We look like such . . . consumers. Wasteful consumers."

"So?" Denis would reply.

"Well, everybody has this impression that Americans are wasteful consumers, and I'd hate for people to think . . ."

"That you're an American?" Denis laughed. "I've got news for you. . . ."

"Maybe I'll start using cloth diapers. I think that's why we have so much garbage," I said.

Denis had to deprogram me in a sense, and he did this by remarking constantly about how inconvenient everything was in England.

"This is a country that is centuries old, whose vast empire once ruled the world. You'd think in all that time they might have been able to come up with a recipe for absorbent toilet paper!" he'd holler from the bathroom.

"Jesus Christ!" he'd say, returning from a late-night gig. "I just took a minicab home, but it was no cab—it was a covered skateboard. I could barely get myself out of the thing."

"It's the twentieth century!" he'd bellow from the shower. "We have the technology to make water come out stronger than a fuckin' trickle. I'm fuckin' freezing in here!"

BY THE TIME the Fourth of July rolled around, I imagined that if I ever did make it back to my beloved homeland, I would sink trembling to my knees and kiss her hallowed earth. On that day I was watching a documentary about Elvis Presley, and he sang a medley that began with "Dixie" and ended with "God Bless America." Although the only southern state I've ever visited is Florida, when Elvis sang "Dixie," my heart ached for the old times there, and by the time the King finished his mournful ballad, I was sobbing. Right around then, Queen Elizabeth was visiting the United States and was taken on a tour of a Philadelphia housing project. The press followed her into the home of one of the residents, who decided that the best way to greet a famous queen was to give her a big ol' bear hug, which sent the queen into a state of shock and was the subject of headlines all over the UK for at least a week. To me the encounter said volumes about British-American relations, and I felt very much like the affable but clueless American woman in the news.

I wanted to go home. I wanted to drink strong cups of

brewed coffee and talk on the phone with my mother about nothing important. I wanted to order a sub or a slice to go and drink lemonade made from real lemons and eat fresh corn on the cob. I wanted to meander down a familiar street with my baby in a stroller and know that there was a possibility I might run into an old friend.

An older English doctor I had met at the hospital told me she'd done one year of college in America. She reminisced about the way she had wanted to be able to walk like American girls. "The way they ambled along, swinging their arms—I really wanted to emulate their uninhibited style, but I couldn't." Now I wanted, more than anything in the world, to go home and move freely and unabashedly like the American girl I used to be. My American, pre-baby self was recalled in my mind now like a dear, departed friend. Like a dead friend, really, and just as we usually retain only rosy memories of our dead friends, when I thought of my former self, it was always in glowing terms. I recalled with loving affection the carefree young girl who loved dogs and horses and dancing at nightclubs and watching old movies. I remembered how I used to walk home to Charlestown on the North End Bridge after work and how I would smile flirtatiously back at the leering longshoremen and construction workers I passed along the way. How I used to wake up on Sunday and buy coffee and the paper on the corner and stop in the local bakery for hot, fresh-baked sticky buns to take back home to Denis. I remembered the summers when Denis would work comedy clubs on the Cape and how the club owners would put us up in fly-infested cabins for a week and we would swim and eat fried clams and drink beer and stay up all night playing gin rummy and then making love. When I was young, I always thought of myself as worldly and wise beyond my years, but now I was a mother, and I saw my former self as I really was—hopelessly innocent and naïve and unfinished, and I desperately wanted to be that way again.

PART FOUR

Auld Reekie

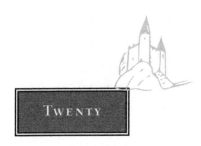

THE EDINBURGH INTERNATIONAL Arts Festival is one of the largest annual arts festivals in the world. It began in 1947, as a postwar effort to reunite the cultural communities of Europe and the United Kingdom. The first festival was so inspired and highly anticipated that there were more performers than venues, so in addition to the promoted, featured performances that year, there were eight uninvited acts that crashed the event in order to take advantage of the crowds and publicity, which is how the Fringe Festival was born. Over the years many famous performers have gotten their start at the Fringe Festival, including John Cleese and Monty Python's Flying Circus, Dudley Moore, and many others. In August 1990 Denis was going to bring his one-man show to the Edinburgh Fringe Festival.

John Thoday, Denis's manager, had him booked into clubs two or three nights a week, but he didn't want Denis on the road too much, as it was only a few weeks until the festival, and he wanted Denis to have time to write. Soon posters began arriving in our flat featuring a huge photo of Denis smoking a cigarette and the title of the show, *No Cure for Cancer,* emblazoned across the front, along with the name of the venue in Edinburgh where Denis was to perform. Denis would wake up in the morning and stare at the posters while he ate his cereal. "I really have to finish writing that show," he'd say calmly, and then he'd wander into the living room and turn on the television.

In 1990 there were only four channels available to most British viewers: BBC1, BBC2, ITV, and Channel 4. This might seem like a meager selection to those who grew up with hundreds of cable channels at their fingertips, but the truth was that almost everything on British television, including the ads, was unbelievably good. Each night there were riveting documentaries, extremely funny comedies, teleplays, quiz shows, and, with amazing frequency, nature programs.

It was almost impossible to turn on the TV that summer and not see a program about small woodland creatures on one of those four channels. Unlike American nature programs, which typically featured sleek tigers and voracious lions, these British documentaries usually centered on voles, weasels, and the ever-popular badger. Badger shows ran constantly. In the morning I would nurse Jack while watching badgers mate. Later Denis would tune in to another channel to find a feature about the nesting habits of badgers. Badgers eating, sleeping, yawning—apparently there was no end to the British appetite for information about these creatures. Although I never saw it, Denis claimed that in the early-morning hours, when most programming was over, one channel showed oddly engrossing footage of badgers with pop music playing softly in the background.

By far our favorite program was *One Man and His Dog*. This was a televised sporting event shown once a week. It was a sheep-herding competition, and each week it took place at a different locale. It was shot on video, and although the camera work was somewhat primitive, the views of the British countryside were beautiful. A small flock of sheep would stand grazing in a meadow. A tweedy old farmer would approach the field with an intensely enthusiastic Border collie. The man would stare at the sheep. The dog, poised for action, would stare at the sheep, then at the man, then the sheep, then the man, the sheep, the man, until finally the man nodded and grunted, and the dog would be off like a low-flying missile aimed right for the sheep. The man would let out a whistle, and the dog would drop to the ground. Another whistle and the dog would crawl along to the left of the sheep or to the right. The dog did all the work, the man stood in one place and whistled orders, and the announcer, in hushed tones, would say things like, "Let's see if Jip can steer them round that last gate . . . oh, *no*! She's lost one! Horrigan must be terribly disappointed with that. She's been a rather unreliable bitch throughout her career, really."

Denis began spending more time writing his show, and I

passed our last few weeks in London walking with Jack through the streets of the city by day and watching television at night. Jack and I would sometimes visit Jo and her daughter, Florence, and occasionally a nurse from UCH would pay us a visit and fill me in on the gossip from the unit.

Denis had asked his friend Chris Phillips to come to the Edinburgh Festival to play the guitar for his show, and Chris arrived in London a few days early, to do a little sight-seeing. Chris's presence distracted us from the surprising melancholy we felt about leaving the city that had held us captive all these months, and it was wonderful to finally be able to show off Jack to an old friend.

During the second week of August, Denis and I packed our few articles of clothing and gave back the books and baby gear we had borrowed from Jo and some of her friends. I phoned Jo and Joan and paid a last teary visit to the neonatal unit at UCH. We had an American passport made for Jack, and in the photo he was held aloft between Denis's hands, his legs dangling like a pup's, his cheeks pink and plump. Finally, on our last morning, we said good-bye to Robert and Brian, Caroline and Sandra, Betty and the loathsome Timmy, and we set off for Edinburgh, Jack snuggled against Denis's chest in his pouch.

The train trip to Edinburgh was very scenic and was really my first glimpse of the British countryside. We had seats that faced each other and a little table between them, where we placed Jack's basket. He obligingly slept most of the way. When he awoke and I nursed him, Chris looked concerned and finally, unable to restrain himself, asked me when I was going to start giving the baby a bottle. I said not for many months, and Chris tried to smile casually, but I could sense his alarm. Later on the trip, Chris warmed up to me to the point where he felt comfortable enough to dispense child-care advice as well as hints regarding how I might make myself more attractive to men. Breast-feeding, I was informed, was going to ruin my breasts and turn Jack into a fag. My decisions regarding feeding and sleeping schedules, burping, and diapering were all scrutinized and basically discredited by this man who had no children and had never dated a woman longer than a few months. Two beautiful, pale children were seated in our car and wandered over from time to time to look at Jack. They asked his name and his age, and because they looked like forlorn English street urchins, Chris would sing a song from *Oliver!*—like "Whe-e-e-re Is Love?"—every time they approached.

The moment we arrived in Edinburgh, a sense of profound relief came over me. The air was cool and crisp and the city more picturesque than I had even imagined. I soon learned that we would be sharing our Edinburgh flat with not only Chris but also Nathan Green, Denis's New York manager. Nathan arrived in Edinburgh with enough luggage to clothe a Scottish regiment, and he and his vast shoe collection took one of the two bedrooms. Denis, Jack, and I took the other, and Chris was required to sleep on the couch in the living room. Chris, it turned out, was not a couch-in-the-living-room kind of guy and fretted constantly about people touching his things. I learned later that he worried incessantly that in the evenings, when he and Denis performed, I might be breast-feeding the baby on the very couch where he slept. As the couch faced the only TV in the place, that's precisely what I was doing. Still, it was a tidy flat, and the building was conveniently located in the old town in the shadow of Edinburgh Castle.

That first evening Denis and I took Jack out for a walk. Despite a light drizzle, the city of Edinburgh was alive. People young and old thronged the streets, and music could be heard all around us. In the parks, in churches and doorways, everywhere, there were jugglers and magicians, portrait artists, gymnasts, and dancers. The crowd that moved along the sidewalks with us was made up of parents and children, junkies and punk rockers, old grannies and hustlers, and tourists of every imaginable ethnicity. And most exciting of all, thanks to the efforts of Denis's brilliant manager, John Thoday, there were posters for *No Cure for Cancer* everywhere we looked. They beamed down at us from the sides of buildings and fences. They adorned streetlights and telephone poles. They were surrounded by hundreds of posters from other shows, but all we could see was Denis, wreathed in smoke, encircled by quotes calling his show "brilliant" and "hilarious."*

---

*These were quotes from British newspapers. Before our trip to London, Denis had received very little notice from the American press, which we considered a blessing, as at the time they had a slightly different perspective on Denis. Most memorable was a *New York Post* review that said, "Denis Leary spread eight seconds of material over what seemed like forty-five days."

Denis reached for my hand, and we strolled along, our little family. Only five months earlier, he and I had walked like this through London, so thrilled at finding ourselves in a strange and exciting city, so completely unaware of the disaster that lay just moments ahead. I had thought of those moments before my PROM thousands of times over the past few months, and when I did, it was like watching a movie in which the subjects don't know they're just about to drive off a cliff or be eaten by a shark. How innocent we were! We had no idea that babies could be born three months early and survive. We had never attended a childbirth class and knew nothing about obstetrics or neonatology. We had only vague, anecdotal ideas of what parenting entailed and not an inkling of the human capacity for hope, despair, fear, desire—the churning, tumultuous, heart-swelling realities of parental love. Somehow we had found our way from that bleak, wet corner on Oxford Street . . . to here! Denis was starring in his own show, which had been successfully previewed in London. There were American and European agents and producers everywhere. It was as if we'd been swept off a beach by a tidal wave that, after dragging us under and smashing our heads against a few rocks, finally tossed us up onto a nicer, more bountiful beach than the one we'd left behind.

Jack's tiny feet dangled from his pouch and bobbed against my belly. From the enclosed fortress of Edinburgh Castle rose the sound of bagpipes, and the smell of wet wool and tobacco smoke and burning peat filled the air around me and I couldn't stop smiling. I cradled Jack's tender feet in my hands, and we followed the crowds through those cobbled Edinburgh roads, the three of us.

AFTER JACK AND I awoke at dawn the next morning, I hastily fed and dressed us both, put Jack in his pouch, and headed out the door to see what I considered to be Edinburgh's most awe-inspiring tourist attraction, Greyfriars Kirkyard, which held a statue of a "wee terrier" named Bobby. Everything I knew about Edinburgh, before that August, I had learned from a Disney movie called *Greyfriars Bobby*.

According to the movie, which I committed to memory as a child, Bobby was a Skye terrier who, sometime during the nineteenth century, belonged to a poor shepherd called "Auld Jock." When Auld Jock died, he was taken to be buried in Edinburgh at Greyfriars Kirkyard. The wee Bobby, who had never left his master's side, followed Auld Jock's body to the kirkyard. Bobby was chased from the kirkyard, but he returned that evening—and every evening for the rest of his life—to lie beside his master's grave. The little dog's fidelity was admired far and wide, and not long after he himself died, a statue of Bobby was erected in the park.

As a young girl, I loved that story and fantasized about having a little dog of my own who would lie shivering on my grave out of absolute devotion to me. In reality I did own a dog—we'd always had dogs when I was a child, but our dogs seemed to be as devoted to the idea of escape as Bobby was to his master, and if we didn't keep them leashed, they would have run off, presumably forever. Bobby, who slept on the ground on a craggy Scottish hillside and was tossed an occasional crust of bread, wouldn't leave his master's side even after his death. Our dogs, who slept in our beds and were fed Alpo Prime Cuts twice a day, viewed themselves as captives and would seek any opportunity to flee. One dog, Coco, in apparent desperation, hurled herself out of our car window as we sped along a country road. So, it was with great admiration that I sought out the grave and monument of the loyal terrier. When we arrived, I managed to prop Jack up against the statue and take his picture.

After paying homage to Bobby, I walked along the High Street and found a coffeehouse. It was not busy inside, just a few hippies and tourists, and the place smelled of clove cigarettes and strong coffee. A cheerful waitress told me to sit where I pleased, and I found a corner table and ordered a coffee and a scone. The coffee was served in a carafe and was so dark and rich I almost wept. The scone was light and flaky, and I smeared it with the freshest, creamiest butter I've ever tasted. Around me I heard German spoken, and French. At the next table, a heavily tattooed man wrote a letter in a surprisingly effeminate hand, and I was suddenly overwhelmed by a sense of belonging. In London I had felt like the guest who wouldn't leave, but here in Edinburgh I felt like a free spirit. The people around me were in Edinburgh to attend the Fringe Festival, a festival in which my husband was performing. No longer the needy losers whose membranes ruptured in other people's countries, we were now an exciting young American family who thought nothing of packing their infant in a little basket and attending arts festivals.

That week Jack and I toured the city each day, only to return to our flat in the evenings, just as Denis and his convoy-in-residence were preparing to leave. From the moment Denis had first mentioned to me the idea of his doing a one-man show at the Fringe Festival, I had viewed the entire idea with skepticism. "A one-man show?" I'd asked. "Who'd want to go see that?" This was to be the first of many, many instances in Denis's career when I was convinced that I was the only person who could see things rationally, who had her finger on the pulse of what an audience will and will not want to see, only to be proved completely clueless and pulseless. Denis's show, which was booked into one of the largest venues at the festival, was sold out the entire week and received outstanding reviews. ("Dazzling. Fearsome. Supremely funny," said the London *Times*.) I couldn't attend any of the shows because I had Jack, but each evening before they left, Denis and Chris would fill me in on some of the highlights from the previous night's show. Then, after being quizzed by Chris about which of his belongings I usually touched while he was out, I would be left alone with Jack to lactate with wanton abandon.

After a few nights of this, I was lonely. I was in a city alive with festivities, and each night, as I watched television documentaries about badgers or voles, I heard the military tattoo performed next door at the castle with its drums and bugles and thunderous cannons. Far into the early-morning hours, laughter could be heard on the streets, and at dawn, when Jack and I were usually ready for our first outing of the day, a stray couple would sometimes still be making their way home, each wearily supporting the weight of the other.

At the time, there were a number of walking tours advertised on posters throughout the city. Tours of churches, gardens, and castles held no real appeal for me, but I found myself stopping several times a day to study a poster boasting the line FEEL THE SPIRIT OF AULD REEKIE in red Gothic lettering. It was an advertisement for a tour of "Haunted Edinburgh." The tour promised to visit the "witching points" where witches had been burned alive and to travel along the cruelly cobbled streets where they had been dragged, again alive, behind carriages. But it was the prospect of an encounter with this mysterious Reekie that captured my imagination. Denis had caught a cold soon after our arrival, and some concerned individual, whom I never got a chance to thank personally, suggested that he drink tea made from raw garlic, which he did, by the pint. Then he would sweat onstage for two hours, drink and smoke with his friends, and by the time he returned to the flat each night, he seemed possessed by something evil indeed. Something that might easily have been mistaken for the spirit of Auld Reekie, so I felt a spiritual connection and was soon consumed by the idea of taking the tour.

I decided to save the tour for our last night in Edinburgh. It was to begin at the "witching hour," which, according to the poster, was 8:30 P.M. As the hour grew near, I fed Jack, bundled him into his pouch, and was just heading out the door when I realized I'd forgotten to ask Denis to leave me the six pounds for the tour. It was now seven-thirty, and Denis was about to go onstage—someplace. I knew that his show was in a theater called the Assembly Rooms, but I had no idea where these Assembly Rooms were. I quickly made my way to the High Street, looking for ads for Denis's show on every wall and lamppost. As is usual in situations like this, Denis's poster, which in the preceding days had beamed down at me on every corner, was now nowhere to be found. I walked for blocks and wandered into various performance halls, but I was usually met at the door by an employee who glared at Jack.

"You're not coming in here with . . . that?" asked one house manager, and the way he scowled at Jack, you'd have thought I had a bomb strapped to my chest.

"Can you please tell me where the Assembly Rooms are?" I asked, but the man had turned away and was taking tickets from the other people in line. It was now eight-twenty, and I was sick with self-pity. The one thing I had looked forward to, I was going to miss. Denis got to do incredibly exciting things every night, but I had only this meager hope for a little fun in Edinburgh, and it had been dashed because my husband was too self-centered to ask me if I needed six pounds before he left. Fighting tears, I began to walk back to our flat, when suddenly I spotted Nathan Green coming toward me.

"Please, Nathan, can I borrow six pounds?" I begged.

"Six quid?" he replied. "Not a problem."

I forced a smile. Nathan had been in the UK for one week and had eagerly adopted every bit of British slang he could wrap his nasal Long Island accent around. Words like "yob," "quid," and "bloke" proudly peppered his conversation now, accompanied by only a vague understanding of the customary usage of the words.

"Thanks," I said to Nathan, and hurried off toward the Royal Mile.

"Cheers!" Nathan called after me.

IT WAS EIGHT-FORTY when we arrived at the Tron, on the Royal Mile, and at the corner where the tour was supposed to meet, there was a kiosk for Edinburgh Walking Tours, but its window was closed. I looked up the road and saw a large group of people following a man in a dramatic top hat and cape. A police officer stood next to the kiosk, and I asked him if that tour had embarked from this corner.

"If it's the ghost tour yer after, that's the one," he replied.

I asked the man if there was someplace I was supposed to pay, and he said that usually people pay at the kiosk, but latecomers could surely pay at the end, and he urged me to hurry up and join them.

So I joined the tour and listened with rapt attention to the guide, who called himself the grand master and high priest of some type of pagan coven. His performance seemed a little forced, as if he'd had a few hundred too many witching hours that summer, but he was periodically relieved from his diatribe by other costumed characters whom we met along the way. For example, turning the corner into a narrow alley, we suddenly encountered a ghoulish creature that leaped out at us and caused me to shriek and then laugh maniacally from nervous excitement. It was the spirit of an unfortunate soul who wanted to share with us her experience of being tortured to death by John Kincaid, the famous "witch pricker." On the next block, Dr. Jekyll peered out a window at us and warned us of a dangerous criminal on the loose, and later Mr. Hyde lunged at us with a bloody knife.

I usually avoid anything that involves audience participation, but that evening I laughed uproariously at the speaker's jokes and recoiled in mock horror at the apparitions that staggered, limped, and cursed at us from various doorways and street corners. I soon worked my way to the front of the crowd, and when the speaker asked literary questions that were so simple even I knew the answer, my hand shot up eagerly. I was having the time of my life. Again, I had this strong sense of belonging. Walking from one attraction to the next, I chatted with some of the other tourists. There was a couple from Brussels and an elderly Englishwoman who asked me Jack's age and then commented on his tiny size. I told her that he had been premature, and she smiled kindly at me and said, "Bless him."

It was late in the day. The sky and the narrow road and old buildings were all a grayish pink in the twilight, and we moved along behind our guide like a contented flock. We ascended a hill, and the city spread below us, and I felt like I'd been there before, right in that very spot on that road built eight hundred years before. My sleeping baby was slung across my chest, and I stood above an ancient city, shoulder to shoulder with my brethren.

We started to move on down the hill when the guide said, "Wait, I almost forgot . . . everybody raise both hands!"

I reached for the sky and was surprised to see that few others did as well.

"Now," said the guide, staring fixedly at me, "I must ask those of you with your hands up to leave this tour. Those who have *paid* have been instructed not to raise both hands—it was worked out at the onset. After all, it's not fair to those who have *paid* to have people just tag along for *free,* is it?"

All eyes were now on me. Instantly I had gone from the most enthusiastic member of the tour to one of the spectacles—an outcast heathen—and I slowly covered Jack's tiny body with my coat. Then, with some sidelong glances and a few smirks, the group moved on, leaving me and a couple of tipsy Germans standing where the group had stood just a moment before. I considered running to the front of the tour and explaining to the guide and the rest of the group that my intention was to pay at the end. I thought of myself waving my money frantically, seeking eye contact with someone—the English lady, anyone who might believe me. But what if nobody did? I stood and watched my group make their way toward . . . who-knew-what. A witch whose skin had been boiled off her body alive? Auld Reekie himself?

The sun had settled below the hills, and it was getting cold. My abrupt stillness had awakened Jack, and now his head moved back and forth, his lips rooting about in the air for sustenance. I kissed his head on the soft spot, still so delicate, so unspeakably vulnerable, and I was filled with tenderness and love. The urgent, primitive longing to nourish and protect was upon me, and I know it sounds trite now, but I felt like Mary then, just full of grace. I helped Jack find his little fist, and he sucked it for a few moments and fell back to sleep, and the ground beneath me, once so foreign and unyielding, was suddenly mine. I turned my back on the departing group—on the trusting fold of tourists and their native-born leader. I buttoned my jacket around my son and started up the Royal Mile toward home.

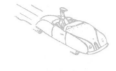

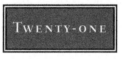

Twenty-one

HEN WE ARRIVED at Logan Airport in Boston the following night, my mother and Steve and my sister, Meg, were waiting. My father and Terry were there also; they'd driven all the way up from Connecticut just to greet us and videotape our arrival. My mother waved a small American flag so that we could see them in the crowd when we came out of the terminal. I had envisioned this moment for months. I had imagined all of us running toward each other in slow motion, tears streaming down our faces, Denis holding Jack aloft for all to see. But I was too exhausted from the flight to feel any emotion, too distracted by the sudden sense of being home and not knowing where I was. Dry-eyed, I hugged my parents and sister, and we climbed into the back of my mother's car, Jack nestled asleep in his car seat.

Several weeks later Denis, Jack, and I moved into a rental apartment building on Manhattan's Upper West Side. It was one of those large white-brick buildings constructed in the 1960s, and it was populated almost exclusively by the elderly. Every day when I wheeled Jack out of the elevator in his stroller, I had to walk through the lobby, which was the roosting spot for all the old resident widows. They took daily outings from their apartments but never ventured past the lobby. In my mind they lay in wait all day for the moment I appeared, so that they could begin their chorus of disapproval.

"Why don't you have a hat on that baby, for heaven's sake? It's not even sixty degrees out, and the wind is gusting," one old biddy would commence, and then they'd all join in.

"My daughter-in-law's the same. Pushing a stroller in a mini-skirt with her bosom exposed for all the world to see. I don't get it. Why advertise when you've got nothing to sell?"

"That's the baby from 6B. The husband doesn't work."

"He works! He works! I saw him come in late one night. I think he's a musician. Or a cabbie."

"The baby wants a bottle. Mama! Your baby's upset. Where's his baba?"

"He's cute, but he doesn't look like the father."

"How would you know? You've never seen the father."

"I saw him. He's black."

"Black? No, Louise, I've told you again and again that's the man from 11C."

"Well, he has a wife. And a baby!"

"A wife and a baby, yes. *This* wife and baby, no."

And they would carry on like this until we left the building. When we first moved in, I would actually try to appease them by adjusting Jack's outerwear to their liking and answering their questions about my personal habits, but slowly I began to ignore them, just as their own children did. I didn't pay attention to what they said, but I secretly loved their very American sense of entitlement to us and to everything else around them. In London people mind their own business. They don't want to embarrass strangers by talking with them, but they're sometimes so insular that they will scurry down into the Underground with eyes shielded, rather than help a woman with a baby stroller down the stairs. New Yorkers will go out of their way to hold open a door or help you carry a stroller, but while doing so, they'll tell you about their sister's fertility problems or ask you how many children you have and why you don't have more.

I was never able to heed Dr. Singh's advice about forgetting Jack's difficult beginning and not making him too precious. Jack was over a year old before I could bring myself to leave him with a sitter, for even an hour or two. My sense of the world had been altered slightly but permanently when Jack was born in the wrong place at the wrong time, and I didn't think any human besides myself was an appropriate caregiver. What if the baby-sitter didn't strap him into his high chair and he fell out? What if he choked? What if the sitter smoked crack cocaine and then threw Jack out the window? The world had changed from a place where anything was possible in a positive sense to one in which anything was possible in a delightful as well as a dreadful sense, and I approached life with a newfound wariness.

Just before Jack's second birthday, his sister, Devin, was born after a full-term pregnancy and a relatively uncomplicated birth, and I began to relax a little bit. I remember walking down Broadway, the four of us, one day in early spring when Devin was just a few weeks old. Denis pushed Jack in his stroller, and I carried Devin across my chest in a pouch, and I was aware of how complete we seemed, our little herd. We walked to the park and ran into a few people we knew. We stopped on a bench to wipe Jack's nose and change Devin's diaper, and then we watched Jack run ahead of us after a pigeon. On the way home, rap music blared from an open car window on Columbus Avenue. The sun had disappeared behind the buildings, and the air was becoming thin and cold. We walked along, and I knew the smells of each block—garbage on one corner, coffee and garlic on the next—and I had a sudden awareness that we were a family, an American family, and New York was our home.

While I was busy birthing and suckling and fretting over our babies, Denis became famous. I had no idea at the time. I think he tried to tell me, but I was too distracted. Jack and Devin and I were doing the "Mommy and Me" circuit all over the Upper West Side. The minute the babies were old enough to support their own heads, they, like many of their tiny New York peers, were enrolled in an exhaustive curriculum of classes to help prepare them for preschool. They began gymnastics and dance classes before they could walk. They took art and music classes before they could hold a spoon. These classes were filled with mothers and caregivers who tumbled and danced and painted and clapped while their babies sat and drooled on the floor. The story hours at the library, the play groups and birthday parties and Gymborees became such an all-consuming whirlwind of activity that although I got to be a first-class tumbler and finger-painter, I lost track of Denis's career.

The year that Devin was born, despite my advice to forget comedy and get a more dependable job writing for television, Denis took his one-man show, *No Cure for Cancer,* Off-Broadway, to the Actors' Playhouse. The show, which had been written only because our baby was too weak to fly, had a sold-out run and produced a book and a bestselling CD. Denis's friend, director Ted Demme, shot some short segments of the show, and they ran constantly on MTV. Denis was also on Comedy Central and HBO regularly, but the only things I ever saw on television in those days were *Barney* and *Sesame Street.*

One night when Devin was a few months old, Denis insisted that I get a sitter. We had been invited to a film premiere at the Ziegfeld Theatre. I can't remember the name of the film, but I'll never forget the shock of having fifty photographers hollering, "DENIS! DENIS, OVER HERE! DENIS LEARY!" as we walked the red carpet leading into the theater.

I clutched Denis's arm in fright. "What do they want? How do they all know your name?" I asked.

Denis said, in a slightly exasperated tone, "I've told you again and again. I'm famous." And we walked out of the dark street right into those blinding lights.

ACK IS NOW thirteen years old. He's the tallest boy in his class and is just teetering on the edge of adolescence, which means that although he knows he's smarter than Denis and me, he still likes us and isn't too embarrassed to bring his friends around. He plays hockey and baseball. He plays the drums. He is a brilliant physical comedian, a master impersonator, and, when he feels like trying, a very good student.

We live in a Connecticut farmhouse now, and not long ago I was in our basement looking for a flashlight and came across a box of photos. Our house is old, and the basement was designed for shorter people. Shorter people who don't mind dirt floors and damp holes in the foundation where mice and snakes creep in. So I grabbed my flashlight and the box and ran upstairs to the kitchen, where I was thrilled to discover that the photos were from the SCBU. I hadn't seen these photos in years, and as I gazed at them one by one, I heard the screen door slam.

"MOM?" Jack called from the front room.

"I'm in the kitchen," I called back.

"I'm . . . [*a string of unintelligible words*], okay?" Jack replied.

"What?" I said.

"I'm . . . [*more gibberish*] Adam's, okay?"

"I'M IN THE KITCHEN! COME IN HERE, PLEASE!" I shrieked.

Jack walked into the kitchen and looked at me like I was insane.

"All right! How come you're yelling?" he said. "Jeesh!"

"You know I don't like yelling from room to room. When you want to speak with somebody, you need to go into the room where they are. I don't know why I have to keep telling you this."

"Oh. Sorry. I'm going to Adam's, okay?"

"Are you walking?"

"No, riding my bike."

"Well, be careful. Stay on the right side of the road."

"I know," Jack said.

"Don't talk to anyone. If somebody slows down to ask directions or something, just ride away. Don't get—"

"Mom, I know."

"All right. Just be careful."

"What're those pictures of?" Jack asked.

"You, when you were a little baby. When you were in the hospital in London."

"Can I see?" said Jack, so I handed him a photo that was taken just a few days after his birth. It showed Jack in his isolette and me sitting next to him, staring dazedly up at the camera. Jack studied the picture and I saw the color drain from his face.

"Don't you remember these photos?" I asked him.

"No," said Jack.

"I used to show them to you when you were younger. They were kind of buried away. I just came across them this afternoon."

Jack continued to stare at the picture, frowning.

"They're kind of hard to look at, aren't they?"

"Kind of?" Jack replied. "You look like a guy with that haircut! Did Dad ever see you like that?"

"Well, of course," I said.

"Did you go out in public like that?"

"Yes . . ."

"Mom, no offense, but . . ."

Now I braced myself. My kids believe that the slap of any insult is somehow soothed by prefacing it with "no offense, but . . ."

"You look like a freak."

Then, trying to placate me with a smile, he handed the photo back and went bounding out of the room with his dog, Rocky, at his side, and I turned my attention back to the photographs.

* * *

JACK'S ONLY PHYSICAL scars from his prematurity are a con-
stellation of tiny white dots on his hands, wrists, and feet.
These are from the many blood tests, transfusions, and IV needles he endured during his time in the unit. You can really only
see them in the summer, when his skin is tan. Today he's proud
of these battle wounds and often asks me to confirm for his
friends that he was indeed two pounds when he was born.
(Thirteen-year-olds consider other thirteen-year-olds lousy
sources and always insist on corroborating stories when being
issued a brag.)

And I have a lingering scar of my own that exists to this day.
Every now and then I'm stricken with an immediate and heart-
wrenching awareness of the prodigious wonder of Jack's existence. I'm sure all parents experience this with their first child,
but I think that during those months in London, I overtaxed the
part of my psyche that inhibits embarrassing public demonstra-
tions of feelings, and I find myself now rendered emotionally
incontinent when it comes to both of my children, but especially Jack. When Denis plopped Jack in Santa's lap at Macy's
that first Christmas, for example, the whole absurdly American
splendor of the moment caught me by surprise and, as six-foot-
tall elves made faces at Jack to get him to smile and "I'll Be
Home for Christmas" was piped at a deafening pitch into my
ears and Jack sought out my face before producing a deliciously

gummy smile, I burst into fitful, sobbing tears and had to be led from Santa's cave supported by two nervous reindeer in mini-skirts.

When Jack was born three months early, I bitterly envied the pregnant women I saw walking down the street. I felt then that my pregnancy had been stolen from me, but now I know that it was Jack's pregnancy, too, not just mine, and it was never really under my control. Having children really is like driving a car from the backseat, without a steering wheel, just like in my childhood nightmares, and sometimes the car simply goes too fast past the things we'd have preferred to stay and enjoy a little bit longer, and we have to keep our eyes open and take in the changing scenery now, knowing we'll never pass this way again. I still meet all of Jack's firsts with the same dizzying emotional confusion of joy, gratitude, wonder, and, of course, sorrow that we've left a part of our lives behind forever. It was this bitter-sweet blend of pride and nostalgic longing that summoned those annoying and embarrassing tears at Jack's christening, his first steps, his first day of school, and the first time, after many weeks of Little League, that he swung his bat in a perfectly timed arc and met the pitched ball with a resounding *thwack,* then paused before running to watch in wonder as his first hit entered the world.

Acknowledgments

First, Denis and I are forever indebted to University College Hospital, London. Without the professional expertise and compassionate care provided by the entire staff, this book might have had a very different ending. In particular, I'd like to thank Mae Nugent, Dr. John Wyatt, Dr. Ann Stewart, Jan Townsend, Mr. Siddle, and all the others whose names I've forgotten but whose kind hearts will always be remembered.

Other Brits and Yanks who were there for us then: Jo Andrews, Heather and Bill Lowden, David Baddiel, Steve and Judy Howe, Meg Seminara, Bill Lembeck, Lindsey Brown, Kristin Johnson, Tony V., Betsy Hilton, Nora Leary, Juliana Nash, Jennifer Blaikie, Ann Marie and Neil Coleman, and John Thoday.

And those who saw me through the year of writing this book:

Paula Gallagher, Paul Healy, Susan Katzenberg, Wendy Burden, Lisa Hedley, Jen Carolan, Donna Zehring, Marc Morgan, my precious children—Jack and Devin, who ate macaroni and cheese three times a week—my agent, Henry Dunow, and my truly remarkable editor, Trish Grader, who helped me make sense of it all.

Very special thanks to my dear friend, the author Heather King, who not only saved my letters from London but offered me lots of encouragement, guidance, and many laughs over the years.

And finally, without the encouragement of Denis Leary, I would never in a million years have written one single word once I finished college. It was only his insistence on referring to me as a writer that shamed me into actually writing something. For this and so many, many other things, I offer my loving gratitude.

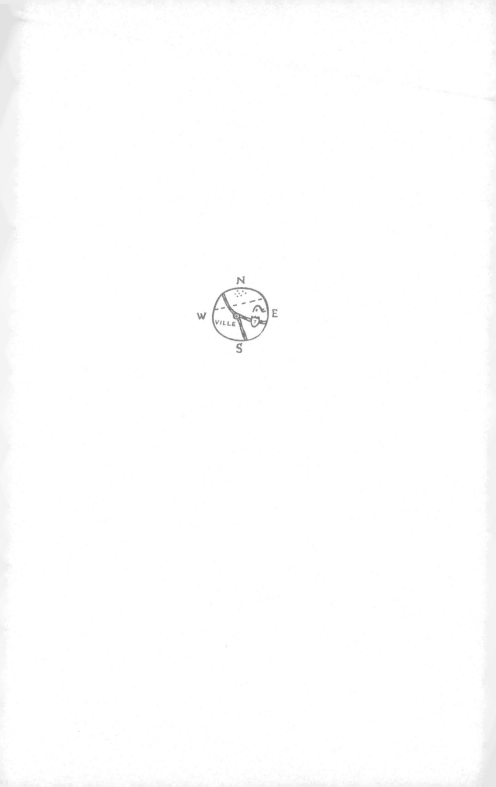

Made in the USA
Monee, IL
22 May 2023

34346179R00152